ALZHEIMER'S DISEASE HANDBOOK

ADVANCES IN THE UNDERSTANDING AND TREATMENT OF ALZHEIMER'S DISEASE AND OTHER DEMENTIAS

CORNELIUS KELLY MB Bch MRCPsych Mphil,

CONSULTANT IN MENTAL HEALTHCARE FOR OLDER PEOPLE,
HOMERTON HOSPITAL, LONDON, ENGLAND

CONTRIBUTORS

FRANCIS BURNETT MB ChB MRCGP MRCPsych
CONSULTANT IN MENTAL HEALTHCARE FOR OLDER PEOPLE,
HOMERTON HOSPITAL, LONDON, ENGLAND

VINCENT KIRCHNER MB ChB FCPsych (South Africa)
SPECIALIST REGISTRAR IN MENTAL HEALTHCARE FOR OLDER PEOPLE,
HOMERTON HOSPITAL, LONDON, ENGLAND

MARTIN VERNON MB MRCP
CONSULTANT GERIATRICIAN, HOMERTON HOSPITAL, LONDON, ENGLAND

ZUZANNA WALKER MD (Prague) MRCS LRCP DGM MRCPsych
SENIOR LECTURER/HONORARY CONSULTANT IN PSYCHIATRY
FOR THE ELDERLY UNIVERSITY COLLEGE,
LONDON MEDICAL SCHOOL AND HERTS & ESSEX COMMUNITY NHS TRUST

MERIT PUBLISHING INTERNATIONAL

European address

1st Floor, 35 Winchester Street,
Basingstoke, Hampshire RG21 7EE,
England
Tel: 01256 841008
Fax: 01256 841099
Email: merituk@aol.com

North American address

8260 NW 49th Manor,
Coral Springs, Florida 33067
USA
Tel: (954) 755 4280
Fax: (954) 755 4287
Email: meritpi@aol.com
www: meritpublishing.com

ISBN: 1 873413 37 8

Disclaimer: This book has been sponsored by an educational grant from Eisai Limited and
Pfizer Limited. The views and opinions expressed are those of the authors and not
necessarily those of either Eisai Limited or Pfizer Limited.

CONTENTS

Introduction

Dementia in the Second Millennium A.D.

Brice Pitt

The Seventh age of man, according to Jacques in *"As you like it"*, is:

> *"Last scene of all, which ends this strange, eventful history is second childishness and mere oblivion; Sans teeth, sans eyes, sans taste, sans everything".*

In Shakespeare's day this may have seemed the inevitable consequence of being so presumptuous as to live too long. Nowadays, however, we have remedies for some of this selection of age-related disabilities: conservative dentistry and dentures leave few old people functionally edentulous, and prostheses for presbyopia, prophylactic drops for glaucoma, enucleation and lens replacement for cataract and laser treatment for detached retina means that few end their lives blind.

However, the spectre of 'senile' dementia has haunted generations before and after Shakespeare's time. We now know that this is not the fate of all who exceed the Biblical 'three score years and ten'; the risk of dementia certainly increases with ageing, but even over the age of 80 it afflicts only one person in five over eighty. For good or ill, though, we do not know who will be affected. Genetic factors are important in early onset dementia, but are not very striking in old age. Obesity, hypertension, diabetes, smoking and excess alcohol consumption are risk factors for vascular disease and thus for vascular dementia, but only the apolipoprotein phenotype E4 indicates those at risk of Alzheimer's Disease, with insufficient predictive value to be of clinical use.

Nevertheless, the statement indicates what a long way we have come in our understanding of dementia in the last 30 years - since it was recognised that the commonest cause of 'senile dementia' is the pathology described by Alois Alzheimer at the beginning of the 20th century. The 'Alzheimerisation' of senile dementia has transformed the attitudes of the scientific community and the general public. What was thought of as an aspect of senility became a disease, to be researched with a view to cure. The rapid ageing of the world's population has made the need for a remedy the more pressing, as health and welfare services are seen as potentially overwhelmed. No major, reputable research institution is now without dementia programmes.

We now understand that Alzheimer's Disease is the commmonest of many dementias (vascular, Lewy body, frontal lobe, Creuzfeld-Jakob, Huntington's being among the important others), and that there is likely to be more than one form of Alzheimer's Disease. Through studies of the susceptibility of central cholinergic neurones, the association with Down's syndrome, the implication of amyloid precursor and tau proteins and the identification of genes responsible for some of the rare familial early onset forms, a picture is starting to take shape from the pieces of the jigsaw puzzle of Alzheimer's Disease. And with understanding comes the hope of effective therapies.

Already logical cholinergic treatments using oral anticholinesterases are showing some efficacy in early cases of Alzheimer's Disease, and attempts are being made to determine what distinguishes those who respond from those who do not. Direct stimulants to muscarinic receptors in post-synaptic neurones may soon be introduced, and the potential of anti-inflammatory drugs, preventing oxidative damages by free radicals, regulating calcium entry to mediate damage from glutamate and inhibiting the enzymes that snip our beta-amyloid peptide from amyloid precursor protein to prevent the formation of amyloid plaques are under scrutiny. It is a gratifying challenge to keep abreast of all that is going on in this exciting, prolific field of research.

Nor are psychological approaches neglected. The protective effects of education are noted in therapy based on the 'use it, don't lose it hypothesis' for dementia in the community in Japan (which has seen the world's greatest rate of ageing in the last 50 years); as yet practice may be ahead of the evidence, and we must recall the rather meagre benefits of reality orientation therapy, but - this is the space to watch!

In the meantime, the development of psychogeriatric services and memory clinics, of community services, of humane and homely nursing homes and above all support for the families who bear the burden of care, will ensure the best deal for sufferers and their carers. The Alzheimer's Disease societies have represented consumers very ably, and have shown expertise in public education and the application of political pressure.

Returning, then, the seventh age of man, we can say to the contemporary Jacques: "Perhaps there's no need to be quite so melancholy! The new millennium will surely see a better prospect than 'mere oblivion'.

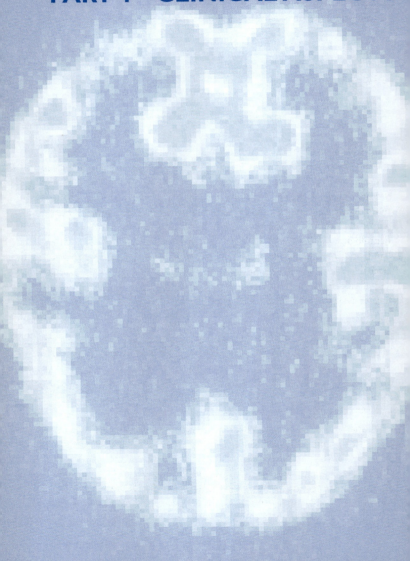

PART 1 - CLINICAL ASPECTS

Chapter 1

Assessment and investigation of dementia

Z Walker

History

The first step when assessing a patient with cognitive difficulties is to obtain a detailed history from the patient and from an independent informant. This point cannot be overemphasised, as is illustrated by the case of a woman in her 60s, who was sent to a neurology clinic with a complaint of inability to use her right hand and a provisional diagnosis of carpal tunnel syndrome. On more detailed questioning the patient's husband mentioned some difficulty with concentration and memory. On examination there were no focal neurological signs but severe apraxia accounted for the inability to use her hand, and she also had severe memory impairment and mild dysphasia. It was clear that the patient's difficulties reflected widespread cognitive impairment, and after initial investigations she was referred to a memory clinic for a further assessment of dementia.

With increased awareness among the general public of the diagnosis of Alzheimer's disease, patients are starting to present to the medical profession in earlier stages of the illness. At the first clinic visit the reason for referral should be established. Is it the patient that is complaining of memory difficulties, or was the referral initiated by a worried relative or other agency e.g. social services? Elderly people who complain bitterly of poor memory are more likely to suffer from depression, anxiety or hypochondriasis than dementia. On the other hand, demented patients frequently lack insight and play down cognitive difficulties they are experiencing. An independent informant in this situation is essential. An opportunity to talk to the carer alone can be very informative as, not surprisingly, there are facts that relatives are reluctant to discuss in front of the patient and they may have worries and issues which they would prefer to discuss without the patient being present.

An attempt should be made to document when problems were first observed, and the type of symptoms that were noticed. Early symptoms are helpful in making an accurate diagnosis. With progression of illness the characteristic deficits which distinguish different types of dementia become less evident and in the end stages all dementias become indistinguishable. It may help informants to date the onset by for instance asking: when did the patient stop sending Christmas or birthday cards, cease to go out and do the shopping, start to need help with bills, forms and appointments. Other enquiries that need to be made include:

Have there been sudden changes in the condition, or has it been a process of insidious onset and progressive decline?

Does the patient's condition fluctuate? Has there been a change in mobility e.g. slowed down, shuffling gait, difficulty getting out of chair or frequent falls? If the answer is 'yes', this raises the possibility of a diagnosis of Dementia with Lewy Bodies (DLB), or vascular dementia or a structural brain lesion.

Is the patient worse at certain times of the day? Being worse in the morning may point to a depressive illness; being worse in the evening raises the possibility of delirium or vascular dementia.

Has there been any change in the patient's interests, hobbies, personality, sexual behaviour, language, ability to do ordinary daily tasks including, using the phone and household equipment?

Can the patient pay in a shop? Are they able to work out the change?

Has there been any change in the patient's self care? Are they losing weight?

Have they recently sustained any injuries or put themselves or others in dangerous situations?

Are they still driving?

Background information about family history of dementia and other neurodegenerative disorders is important. Fifty percent of patients with late-onset AD (Alzheimer's Disease) have a family history of dementia. The presence of a family history, not only of mental illness but also of cerebrovascular disease, diabetes and epilepsy should be established.

Personal history with emphasis on number of years of schooling and professional achievements gives some indication of patient's pre-morbid capabilities and helps to highlight any decline during the early stages of illness.

Establishing previous psychiatric and medical history is essential. Patients should be specifically asked about strokes, heart attacks, diabetes, high blood pressure, major head trauma, epilepsy, central nervous system infections e.g. meningitis, encephalitis. Recurrent depressive episodes in the past raises the possibility of a current depressive illness. Knowledge of the patient's present medication and who, if anybody, is administering or supervising the correct use of prescribed drugs is essential. Finally, inquiries about smoking habits and alcohol intake need to be made. For more detailed reading see, *Psychiatric examination in Jacoby & Oppenheimer, Psychiatry in the elderly*.[1]

Mental state

Appearance and behaviour can sometimes be more helpful in making a diagnosis of dementia than information given by the patient themselves. Appropriateness of clothes for the season and the occasion, their cleanliness, signs of neglected personal hygiene, incontinence and signs of poor nutrition, are all good indicators of how a patient is managing. Aspects of a patient's appearance can give an indication of the chronicity of the disorder, e.g. long and dirty hair and fingernails, ingrained dirt in skin, poorly fitting clothes.

Severe dehydration and fever, breathlessness tachypnoea, tachycardia, swollen legs, clouded consciousness, weakness of one side of the body or dysarthria, should alert the clinician to the possibility of a physical illness and these features may warrant first an assessment/admission by a geriatrician rather than an old age psychiatrist.

Perplexity, restlessness, wandering, repetitive purposeless activity and abnormal movements are observed in more severe cases of dementia. Language can be superficially well preserved in AD and misleading in a short interview, but nominal dysphasia, misuse of words (paraphasias; e.g. lunch for supper, hand for foot, sister for sitter), poverty of detail, polite evasiveness, repetition of themes and inability to take in logical arguments, should alert to the possibility of cognitive impairment.

Suspiciousness, overvalued ideas or delusions and hallucinations are all common in dementia but well formed, persistent visual hallucinations are characteristic of DLB. It is essential to establish the patient's understanding of their illness and their insight into their abilities to manage their affairs, as this has implications for further management.

Great care has to be taken not to confuse deafness, acute confusion, anger, irritability, anxiety, depression or psychosis with cognitive impairment. A considerable amount of information can be obtained from an informal interview with patient and carer but this should be always supplemented with a more formal type of cognitive testing. Even a few simple tests can be amazingly revealing about the extent of the cognitive deficit not only to the doctor but also to the carer.

Cognitive testing

The majority of patients find cognitive testing quite acceptable, particularly if reassured that this is a standard procedure performed by all patients. To be able to perform any formal testing one obviously needs a patient who can co-operate and sustain a degree of concentration and effort, even if this requires a fair amount of encouragement throughout the assessment. Observation of behaviour during the testing is part of the assessment.

There are numerous brief cognitive tests. As the most widely used test is the Mini Mental State Examination[2] (*Table 1*), it will be discussed in more detail. It is a short (5-10 minutes), easily administered scale with a high inter-rater reliability. The maximum score is 30. Scores below 24 are traditionally taken as indicative of cognitive impairment. However, there is a grey area of scores of 24-28 where adjustment needs to be made for age, education and socio-economic status.

This means that in a 70-year-old retired school teacher, a score of less than 28 on MMSE would raise the possibility of an early cognitive impairment. On the other hand, a score of 24, for an 80-year-old woman with only eight years of education, who has been a housewife her whole life, may be acceptable. The most sensitive items on the MMSE for AD are delayed recall of three items and orientation. In patients with high pre-morbid intelligence, a recall of three items can be too easy and should be supplemented with recall of a name and an address (maximum five points).

The MMSE is insensitive for frontal lobe deficit. When fronto-temporal dementia is suspected, additional simple tests of frontal lobe function need to be performed. An easy test to administer is a test of verbal fluency for categories. In this test, the patient is asked to name as many animals as they can in one minute. Less than 15 animals in an elderly patient is abnormal, although, for very old, ten may be just acceptable. In a test of verbal fluency for letters, the patient is asked to produce as many words as possible (excluding names), starting with the letter F in one minute. The same is repeated with the letters A and S. A total for F, A and S of less than 30 is abnormal. Another frontal lobe test is the elucidation of the meaning of proverbs. This can give some indication of a deficit in abstract thinking, as patients with impaired frontal lobe function may give 'concrete' explanations. The ability to explain similarities and differences between two paired items gives some indication of the ability to conceptualise and categorise. For example, ask the patient to say in what way an apple and a banana, or a ship and a train are similar, or ask what the difference is between a mistake and a lie or a canal and a river.

A recent study of 'obstinate imitation behaviour', suggested that this could be a good test to distinguish AD from Front Temporal Dementia (FTD). In this test, the doctor sits opposite the patient and performs a series of gestures ('victory' sign, thumbs up sign, clapping, military salute). If the patient imitates the gestures they are asked clearly not to do so. The doctor than repeats the gestures. If the patient continues to imitate the gestures the test is positive, suggesting that the patient is more likely to suffer from FTD than AD.[3]

The naming of a pencil and a watch in MMSE is not sensitive enough to detect early nominal dysphasia. Showing a patient a wrist watch and then asking them to name the strap, winder, hands and face is more likely to detect a deficit.

Patients with DLB have particular difficulty with copying intersecting pentagons (*Table 1*). This test can be supplemented by testing skills at drawing a clock face. Both patients with AD and DLB have difficulty in drawing a clock with the hands set at 11:10, but DLB patients are even worse than AD patients when asked simply to copy a clock.

One of the most sensitive tests for early AD is the recall of complex verbal information. This can be tested by reading a story (one paragraph), to a

Clinical Report on Ageing

VOLUME 1. NUMBER 1. 1997

Mini-Mental State Examination

Patient's Name: _____ Patient No. _____

Examiner's Name: _____ Date: _____

Patient Score	Maximum Score	
____	5	**Orientation** What is the (year) (season) (date) (day) (month)?
____	5	Where are we (country) (state) (county) (city) (clinic)?
____	3	**Registration** Name three objects, allotting one second to say each one. Then ask the patient to name all three objects after you have said them. Give one point for each answer. Repeat them until he hears all three. Count trials and record number. APPLE TABLE PENNY Number of trials
____	5	**Attention and Calculation** Begin with 100 and count backward by 7 (stop after five answers): 93, 86, 79, 72, 65. Score one point for each correct answer.
____	3	**Recall** Ask the patient to repeat the object above (See Registration). Give one point for each correct answer.
____	2	**Language** **Naming:** Show a pencil and a watch and ask the patient to name them.
____	1	**Repetition:** Repeat the following: 'No ifs, ands, or buts'.
____	3	**Three-Stage Command:** Follow the three-stage command, 'Take a paper in your right hand; fold it in half; and put it on the table.'
____	1	**Reading:** Read and obey the following. 'Close your eyes' (show patient the item written on reverse side).
____	1	**Copying:** Copy the design of the intersecting pentagons (on reverse side).
____	30	Total score possible.

Q6 - Reading

CLOSE YOUR EYES

Q6 - Writing

_____

Q8 - Construction

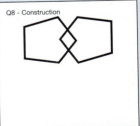

Table 1

patient and asking them to recall everything that they can remember. Recall is again tested after a delay of 20 minutes without prior warning. This test has been derived from the Logical Memory Subtest of the Wechsler Memory Scale. Usually, two stories are used. A healthy elderly patient should be able to recall approximately 25% of the elements of the story, and retain a 55-60% of these after a delay of 20 minutes. In early cases little deficit might be apparent and a more thorough testing by a neuropsychologist, or serial testing will need to be performed. For further reading see *Cognitive assessment for clinicians, Hodges.*[4]

Physical examination

In addition to a standard physical examination special emphasis should be given to some aspects of the neurological examination. Visual fields defects can be easily missed in a patients with dementia. After checking acuity, the visual fields of the two eyes together and of each eye separately should be checked and visual inattention can be looked for at the same time. This might need some persistence from the examiner as patients sometimes find it difficult to comprehend what is asked of them. Homonymous field defects or visual inattention do not occur in AD, and make a diagnosis of cerebrovascular disease or brain tumour likely.

Abnormal eye movements, specifically a selective deficit of vertical gaze, raise the possibility of progressive supranuclear palsy (or an upper brain-stem and thalamic stroke).

The presence of primitive reflexes (grasp reflex, pouting reflex), indicate loss of inhibition from the frontal cortex. Primitive reflexes are commonly found in FTD and DLB, but are also present in normal pressure hydrocephalus, vascular dementia and end stages of AD. They can be present in very old normal individuals and overall are pretty non-specific but do alert clinicians to the presence of an 'organic' disorder.

Signs of hemiparesis, hemianaesthesia or sensory inattention suggest a diagnosis of cerebrovascular disease or a space occupying lesion.

Increased tone in the limbs is either due to neuroleptic medication or raises the possibility of DLB, as does bradykinesia and tremor in the early stages of a dementing illness.

Finally, an examination of the gait is vital in any demented patient. Difficulty rising from a seat without the support of arms, hesitation on starting to walk, a shuffling gait and lack of arm swinging, again point to DLB. On the other hand, an apraxic gait is common in advanced AD and DLB. The gait disorder in vascular dementia is one of apraxia ('marche a petit pas'; 'lower body Parkinsonism'). Normal pressure hydrocephalus is characterised by an ataxic and apraxic gait. Persistently bumping into objects on one side gives a suspicion of visual defect or neglect.

Investigations

There is universal agreement that the initial assessment of a dementia syndrome should comprise history, physical examination, mental state examination and basic neuropsychological testing. However, there continues to be debate about the value of additional investigations in the management of dementia syndromes. There are three questions that need to be answered. First, will further investigations help to identify reversible causes of dementia? Second, will they increase the diagnostic accuracy of different dementia subtypes? Third, will they alter the further management of the patient?

Most clinicians agree that laboratory blood tests are relatively inexpensive and that the cost is justified in every patient with dementia syndrome. *Chui & Zhang* [5] showed that the addition of laboratory tests to the evaluation of dementia changed the diagnosis in 9% and the management in 12.6% of cases. The basic blood tests that should be performed are listed in *Table 2*.

LABORATORY ASSESSMENT FOR DEMENTIA

Full blood count

Erythrocyte sedimentation rate

Serum B_{12} & Folate

Electrolytes, serum creatinine

Glucose

Liver function tests

Calcium

Thyroid function tests

Syphilis serology

Table 2

The routine use of brain imaging remains contentious. MRI is the preferred investigation in dementia but not all clinicians have access to MRI and it is more expensive than CT. CT scans are also better tolerated by demented patients. The main aim is to exclude other intracranial pathology, e.g. primary brain tumours, secondaries, chronic subdural haematomas, infarcts, and hydrocephalus. Neuroimaging is essential for diagnosing Vascular Dementia (VaD) according to the NINDS/AIREN criteria[21]. It is helpful in FTD where it shows preferential fronto-temporal atrophy.

Occasionally, other tests are indicated. EEG may be a valuable investigation in FTD where it remains normal even in more advanced disease. EEG is also helpful in excluding non-convulsive status epilepticus as a complication of dementia. EEG helps in the diagnosis of Creutzfeldt-Jakob disease.

Perfusion single photon emission tomography is particularly useful in the differential diagnosis of FTD, where it shows a characteristic fronto-temporal perfusion defect, compared with a mainly temporo-parietal hypoperfusion in AD.

Lumbar puncture for cerebrospinal fluid analysis is performed very rarely. The main indication is a suspicion of primary central nervous system vasculitis or a paraneoplastic syndrome. In exceptional circumstances, where a treatable cause of dementia is suspected (e.g. primary CNS vasculitis), a brain biopsy may be performed.

References

1. Oppenheimer C, Jacoby R. Jacoby R, Oppenheimer C, editors.Psychiatry in the elderly. Oxford: Oxford University Press; 1991; 7a, Psychiatric examination. p. 169-98.

2. Folstein MF, Folstein SE, McHugh PR. 'Mini-Mental State' A practical method for grading the cognitive state of patients for the clinician. Journal of Psychiatric Research 1975; 12:189-98.

3. Shimomura T, Mori E. Obstinate imitation behaviour in differentiation of frontotemporal dementia from Alzheimer's disease. Lancet 1998; 352:623-4.

4. Hodges JR. Cognitive assessment for clinicians. Oxford: Oxford University Press; 1994; Testing cognitive function at the bedside. p. 108-54.

5. Chui HC, Zhang Q. Evaluation of dementia: A systematic study of the usefulness of the American Academy of Neurology's practice parameters. Neurology 1997; 49:925-35.

Chapter 2

The clinical features of Alzheimer's Disease

C Kelly

Alzheimer's Disease (AD), is the most common cause of dementia, accounting for 50-70% of all cases. The insidious onset and the gradual, but relentless deterioration in cognitive and functional skills, are almost pathognomonic of the condition. Historically clinicians have recognised three phases - early, middle and late - in the progression of the disease. The commonly accepted features of each are given in *Table 3*.

COMMON STAGE-RELATED FEATURES OF ALZHEIMER'S DISEASE

EARLY

Absent minded, difficulty recalling names/words

Increasing forgetfulness

Difficulty learning new information

Disorientation in unfamiliar surroundings

Minor but uncharacteristic lapses in judgement and behaviour

Reduction in social activities both in and out of the home

MIDDLE

Obvious loss of cognitive skills - marked memory loss

Deterioration in verbal skills, range and content of speech diminishes

Increasing behavioural disturbance characterised by: frustration, impatience, restlessness, verbal or physical agression

Obvious decline in social skills

Emergence of psychotic phenomena - paranoid delusions, hallucinations

ADVANCED

Speech becomes monosyllabic and later disappears

Fleeting psychotic symptoms - often because of super-imposed delirium

Behavioural and emotional disturbance

Loss of bladder and bowel control

Mobility deteriorates with shuffling gait, involuntary movements

---

Table 3

Increasingly however, with better assessments and more robust longitudinal data, individual variation is acknowledged, with concomitant variation in brain pathology. Recent research examining the **evolution of psychiatric symptoms in AD**, suggests that the symptom profile may be affected by a number of factors including, gender, age of onset and years of formal education. The medical records of one hundred randomly selected autopsy-confirmed AD cases were retrospectively reviewed for the presence of 16 psychiatric symptoms.[6] A time density plot was constructed to demonstrate a relationship between the frequency and time course of the symptoms. Social withdrawal, occurring 33 months before diagnosis, was the earliest recognisable psychiatric symptom followed by depression, suicidal ideation, paranoia, diurnal rhythm disturbance and anxiety symptoms (*Figure 1*). Patients with more than 12 years of education showed social withdrawal earlier (mean = 30 months), compared with those with less education (mean = 10 months, p=0.055). In general, however, they showed other psychiatric symptoms later, indicating some support for the cognitive reserve theory of education and the expression of

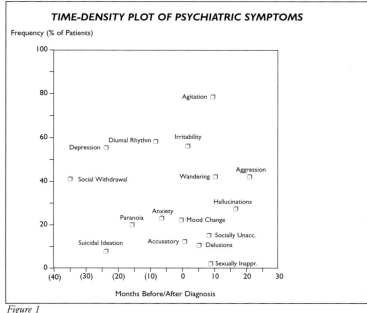

Figure 1

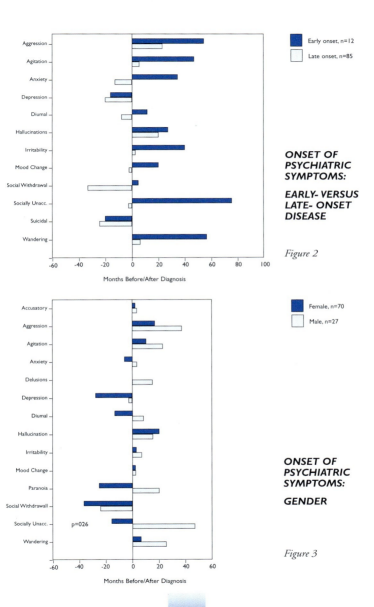

ONSET OF PSYCHIATRIC SYMPTOMS:

EARLY- VERSUS LATE- ONSET DISEASE

Figure 2

ONSET OF PSYCHIATRIC SYMPTOMS:

GENDER

Figure 3

symptoms in AD. Males tended to show psychiatric symptoms later in the course of the disease compared to females (*Figure 2*). Wandering, agitation and aggression were demonstrated significantly later in the course of the disease for early versus late-onset cases (*Figure 3*).

Over the course of the disease, agitative symptoms were documented in 81% of cases, depressive symptoms in 72%, psychotic symptoms in 45% and wandering in 43%. These figures clearly indicate the relevance of psychiatric skills in the assessment and management of AD.

The rate of progression of cognitive and functional decline of patients with AD, was in the past, thought to be generally predictable with characteristic patterns of loss at each stage (*Table 3*). Longitudinal data[7, 8] published in recent years has suggested that a number of factors may predict faster decline; these include older age at onset, disease severity at initial examination, language impairment, extra-pyramidal signs, psychoses and a history of alcohol abuse. While rates of cognitive and functional decline are significantly correlated, particularly in the early years, research increasingly suggests that the processes involved in each may be parallel but distinct. Faster cognitive decline has been demonstrated in patients with poor performance on tests of verbal skills, as well as aggressive behaviour and sleep disturbance, early on in the disease. The rate of functional decline appears to be greater in those with paranoid behaviour, hallucinations and impairment in activities of daily living in the first year and extra-pyramidal signs at the time of specialist diagnosis. The current data therefore suggest that there is no typical rate of progression in either the cognitive or functional domain. As functional decline largely predicts the burden of care, the factors associated with more rapid deterioration should be evaluated and monitored, to optimise care.

Pre-clinical cognitive markers

With the availability of cognitive enhancing treatments, the pre-clinical cognitive markers of AD are increasingly of interest. In particular, it is argued that people with a family history of AD should be screened for cognitive change and those affected, targeted with these treatments in the expectation of delaying conversion to AD. The overwhelming impression from recent research published in this area[9,10,11] is that evidence of verbal memory impairment is the earliest sign of subsequent AD. Detection of verbal memory impairment requires standardised neuro-psychometric testing as AD remains relatively rare whereas 50-80% of elderly people complain of memory loss.

References:

6. Jost BC, Grossberg GT. The evolution of psychiatric symptoms in Alzheimer's disease: a natural history study. J Am Geriatr Soc 1996; 44:1078-1081.

7. Mortimer JA, Ebbitt B, Jun SP, Finch MD. Predictors of cognitive and functional progression in patients with probable Alzheimer's disease. Neurology 1992; 42:1689-1696.

8. Stern Y, Hesdorffer D, Sano M, Mayeux R. Measurement and prediction of functional capacity in Alzheimer's disease. Neurology 1990; 40:8-14.

9. Dartigues JF, Commenges D, Letteneur LD et al. Cognitive predictors of dementia in elderly community residents. Neuroepidemiology 1997; 16:29-39.

10. Bondi MW, Monsch AU, GalaskoD, et al. Preclinical markers of dementia of the Alzheimer type. Neuropsycholgy 1994; 3:374-384.

11. Howieson DB, Dame A, Camicioli R, et al. Cognitive markers preceding Alzheimer's disease in the healthy oldest old. Journal of the American Geriatric Society 1997; 45:584-589.

Chapter 3
Differential diagnosis of Alzheimer's Disease

Z Walker

There are two main questions that have to be answered when assessing a patient with a 'dementia syndrome'. One, is this a true dementia, defined as cognitive impairment in multiple domains with intact arousal and in the majority of cases non-treatable and progressive, or, is this another, possibly treatable, condition mimicking a dementing illness? Two, given that it is a dementia, which type is it? The difficulty is, that a definitive diagnosis of AD, or other dementias, e.g. vascular dementia (VaD), dementia with Lewy bodies (DLB), can only be made at an autopsy. Even then a fair proportion of patients are found to have mixed pathologies. To complicate matters further, there remain unresolved issues about the pathological classification of all the main dementias. The two conditions that most frequently overlap with AD are VaD and DLB.[12] Despite these difficulties, the diagnostic accuracy of AD is no worse (50-90%), than the accuracy of other neuro-degenerative disorders, e.g. Parkinson's disease.[13] The main conditions that need to be considered in the differential diagnosis of AD are listed in *Table 4*.

DIFFERENTIAL DIAGNOSIS OF ALZHEIMER'S DISEASE

Pseudodementia

Delirium

Vascular dementia

Dementia with Lewy bodies

Fronto-temporal dementia

Endocrine and Metabolic disorders

Toxic and Drug encephalopathies

Alcohol related dementia

Normal pressure hydrocephalus

Chronic subdural haematoma

Infectious disease

Creutzfeldt-Jakob disease

Table 4

Depressive pseudodementia

Severe depressive illness with associated cognitive impairment is probably the commonest reversible 'dementia syndrome'. Despite some controversy about the term pseudodementia, in clinical practice it succinctly communicates that the 'dementia syndrome', is not due to a degenerative brain disorder, but is part of a depressive illness and that vigorous treatment of depression is indicated.[13] The features that favour depressive cognitive impairment are complaints by the patient themselves that their memory and concentration is poor, a relatively short history and the patient's ability to date accurately the onset of symptoms. Depressed patients may deny that they are depressed but their whole outlook tends to be negative with no hope or interest in the future and diminished initiative to socialise. Conversation, and in particular, formal cognitive testing, is an effort and 'don't know' answers are more likely than mistakes. Other features pointing to depression are, disturbed sleep, poor appetite, low energy and pessimistic thoughts. There may be a past personal or family history of depression. On cognitive testing there is poor concentration and memory, but with repeated trials there is clear improvement on memory tasks, if the patient can be persuaded to cooperate. Compared with AD, speech is slow and scanty but nominal dysphasia is unusual. Despite the above, it is sometimes impossible to differentiate depressive pseudodementia from dementia with depressive symptoms and only a therapeutic trial with an antidepressants and/or ECT with a longitudinal follow-up settles the matter. One further caveat is that there is evidence that, despite the initial reversibility of cognitive impairment, a higher than expected proportion of patients with depressive pseudodementia go on to develop true dementia.[14]

Delirium

Delirium is now the accepted term for what used to be called 'acute confusional state'. It is defined as an acute, transient, global, organic disorder of higher nervous system function involving impaired consciousness and attention. Delirium carries a significant mortality rate, particularly in the elderly.[15] It is one of the most frequently missed diagnoses in the elderly, patients with delirium being misdiagnosed as having dementia and therefore missing out on appropriate treatment.[16] However, pre-existing dementia is, with advanced age, one of the main risk factors for delirium, highlighting the difficulty of distinguishing the two conditions. Delirium is the result of a primary cerebral disorder or a cerebral involvement secondary to a systemic illness.

The main clinical symptoms are, acute onset, impaired consciousness, reduced ability to maintain attention, disorganised thinking and memory impairment, in particular, registration and retention of new material. Perceptual distortions, leading to misidentification, illusions and hallucinations, and disturbed, sleep-wake cycle are also common. Other symptoms include, mood changes and tendency to fluctuation with occasional lucid period.[17] A history from an informant is the key to the diagnosis. The speed of onset of symptoms (hours, days compared with weeks, months in AD), is one of the main clues to the diagnosis. Consciousness and attention remain unaffected in early stages of AD, whereas in delirium a deficit is present from the start. Delirium can be diagnosed in a known demented patient; on the other hand, if a patient is delirious an additional diagnosis of dementia cannot be made until the delirium has resolved or corroborative history is obtained. However, a known patient with dementia with sudden deterioration in consciousness and attention cannot be automatically assumed to suffer from delirium, as there are other causes of reduced consciousness in a patient with dementia, e.g. sedative medication.

Vascular dementia

The existence of pure vascular dementia (VaD), long regarded as the second most common type of dementia,[18] is now being challenged with researchers and clinicians emphasising the relationship between vascular factors and AD.[18,28] VaD is a broad term that refers to any dementia resulting from cerebral blood vessel disease. This includes, multiple infarcts, strategically placed isolated infarcts, multiple subcortical lacunar infarcts, single or multiple haemorrhagic cerebral lesions, genetically determined arteriopathies, and combined pathologies of AD and infarcts.[17] The main reason for attempting to distinguish VaD from AD was that there were differences in the management of the two conditions. A major aim in patients with VaD was the prevention of further damage to the brain by controlling known risk factors for stroke (hypertension, atrial fibrillation, cigarette smoking, diabetes mellitus and hypercholestrolaemia), and by initiating treatment with small doses of aspirin.[19] It is now recognised that controlling these risk factors is equally important in patients with AD. Cholinesterase inhibitors are only indicated if a mixed pathology is suspected, ie Alzheimer's disease in addition to vascular dementia, although acetyl choline has been shown to play an important role in regulating cerebral blood flow,[20] and clinical trials are underway to test the efficacy of cholinesterase inhibitors in VaD.

The clinical course and the symptoms of VaD vary greatly according to the sites of ischaemia (or haemorrhage), and the type of underlying cerebrovascular disease (CVD). Differentiation between AD and VaD can only be achieved by combining clinical, laboratory and imaging information about a patient. Traditionally, patients with VaD have evidence of focal and non-localising neurological signs attributable to CVD (e.g. dysphasia, dysarthria, hemiparesis, extensor plantar responses and a wide-based small step gait), stroke risk factors, a history of abrupt onset, stepwise deterioration and a fluctuating course of illness. Vascular lesions are identified by neuroimaging, either as single strategic usually cortical infarcs, or multiple infarcts which may be cortical or subcortical. Hypodensities on CT scan in white matter, or hyperintensities in white matter on T_2 weighted MRI, are not easy to interpret and are not very good predictors of VaD, since they are also associated with normal ageing, and with a number of apparently non-vascular dementias including AD. Perfusion studies with Single Photon Emission Tomography (SPET), show irregular deficits, by comparison with the more uniform temporo-parietal hypoperfusion seen in AD. On neuropsychological testing, patients with VaD have a more patchy cognitive deficit and a better preserved insight and personality than patients with AD. Emotional lability and depression are more common in VaD than in AD. VaD has an earlier onset of disease than AD and there is a predominance of males. Of the available criteria,[21] the National Institute for Neurological Disorders and Stroke (NINDS/AIREN), are the ones most commonly used in research settings, although their sensitivity (0.58), is not as good as their specificity (0.80).[22]

Dementia with Lewy bodies

DLB is one of the main differential diagnoses of AD. Autopsy studies have shown that up to 20% of patients with DLB are misdiagnosed as having AD during life. The most characteristic pathological finding in DLB is intraneuronal eosinophilic inclusions - Lewy bodies - in the cerebral cortex. Lewy bodies have been classically associated with Parkinson's disease where they are found mainly in the brain stem. Although 'pure' cortical Lewy body disease exists, the majority of cases have a degree of coexisting Alzheimer's pathology. This presumably explains why the two conditions can be so hard to differentiate clinically. Retrospective analyses of autopsy cases have led to the formulation of consensus criteria for DLB,[23] and prospective studies are in progress to validate these criteria.

Typically, patients with DLB have progressive dementia, although persistent severe memory impairment is not essential in the early stages, compared to AD, where the first feature is always impairment in episodic memory. Prominent deficits in attention, frontal and visuo-spatial ability are more obvious in early DLB. A fluctuating cognitive state with periods of worsening confusion and persistent visual hallucinations, particularly of animals and children, are typical in patients with DLB and unusual in AD. Patients exhibit motor features of Parkinsonism and have repeated unexplained falls. They have frequent adverse reactions to both conventional and atypical neuroleptic drugs.[24,25] Psychotic and behavioural symptoms are common in the later stages and present a considerable challenge to health professionals and carers. Males are more frequently affected. As in AD, the presence of apolipoprotein Ɛ4 alleles is a risk factor for DLB. Various imaging techniques are being assessed to establish their usefulness in differentiating DLB from AD, but at present, no routinely performed investigations have been shown to be helpful.

Fronto-temporal dementia

This is a collection of primary lobar degenerative dementias of non-Alzheimer's type. A number of conditions can be included under this heading. Fronto-temporal dementia (FTD), with and without Pick's pathology (Pick cells, Pick bodies), progressive aphasic syndromes including, semantic dementia and frontal lobe dementia with motor neurone disease. The predominant cortical damage is in the frontal, fronto-temporal, temporal and anterior cingulate gyrus, as opposed to the mainly temporo-parietal and posterior cingulate gyrus pathology of AD.

Consequently, the main clinical features are of frontal lobes dysfunction. In FTD, the characteristic clinical features are striking change in affect, personality and social behaviour, with loss of insight, rapidly leading to inability to manage both at work and also in personal affairs. With disease progression, patients become either withdrawn and apathetic or disinhibited, restless and inattentive. Speech becomes more repetitive and stereotypic, with echolalia and simple songs and rhymes, finally leading to a mute state. Stereotypic and ritualistic behaviours are common, with hyperorality and food fads. Compared with patients with AD, memory and spatial functions are spared, at least in the first few years of illness. However, despite the relatively well-preserved memory, patients with FTD have severe impairment of mental flexibility, organisational skills and abstract thinking.

Occasionally, patients with AD can have an atypical presentation with a frontal lobe syndrome. In these cases, the presence of widespread cognitive deficits, including impairment of episodic memory and visuo-spatial functions from the start of the illness, points to a diagnosis of AD. Clinical and neuropathological criteria for fronto-temporal dementia have been published by the Lund and Manchester groups.[26]

The onset of illness in FTD is earlier than in AD, usually between 45-60 years, with a relatively better survival than in AD, around 10-15 years. Men and women appear to be equally affected. In about half of the patients, an autosomal dominant mode of inheritance has been observed and there is some evidence linking the disease to chromosome 17. The Apolipoprotein ϵ4 allele does not seem to be a significant genetic risk factor for FTD.[27] A normal EEG, despite advanced disease supports the diagnosis. CT or MRI show, at least in some patients, preferential atrophy of the frontal and temporal lobes[28]. A helpful investigation is perfusion SPET, which reveals marked hypoperfusion of the frontal and temporal lobes compared with the characteristic temporo-parietal hypoperfusion of AD.

References

12. Gorelick PB, Nyenhuis DL, Garron DC, Cochran E. Is vascular dementia really Alzheimer's disease or mixed dementia? Neuroepidemiology 1996; 15:286-90.

13. Hughes AJ, Daniel SE, Kilford L, Lees AJ. Accuracy of clinical diagnosis of idiopathic Parkinson's disease: a clinico-pathological study of 100 cases. Journal of Neurology, Neurosurgery and Psychiatry 1992; 55:181-4.

14. Alexopoulous GS, Young RC, Meyers BS. Geriatric depression: Age of onset and dementia. Biological Psychiatry 1993; 34:141-5.

15. Taylor D, Lewis S. Delirium. Journal of Neurology, Neurosurgery and Psychiatry 1993; 56:742-51.

16. Fairweather DS. Jacoby R, Oppenheimer C, editors.Psychiatry in the elderly. Oxford: Oxford University Press; 1991; 18, Delirium. p. 647-75.

17. Nejo TA, Pitt BM. Delirium in elderly people. Current Opinion in Psychiatry 1995; 8:246-51.

18. Loeb C, Meyer JS. Review article - Vascular dementia: still a debatable entity? Journal of the Neurological Sciences 1996; 143:31-40.

19. Gorelick PB. Status of risk factors for dementia associated with stroke. Stroke 1997; 28:459-63.

20. Scremin OU, Jenden DJ. Cholinergic control of cerebral blood flow in stroke, trauma and aging. Life Science 1996; 58(22):2011-8.

21. Roman GC, Tatemichi TK, Erkinjuntti T, et al. Vascular dementia: diagnostic criteria for research studies. Report of the NINDS-AIREN International Workshop. Neurology 1993; 43:250-60.

22. Gold G, Giannakopoulos P, Montes-Paixao C, Herrman FR, Mulligan R, Michel JP, Bouras C. Sensitivity and specificity of newly proposed clinical criteria for possible vascular dementia. Neurology 1997; 47:690-4.

23. McKeith IG, Galasko D, Kosaka K, Perry EK, Dickson DW, Hansen L, Salmon DP, Lowe J, Mirra SS, Byrne EJ, et al. Consensus guidelines for the clinical and pathologic diagnosis of dementia with Lewy bodies (DLB): report of the consortium on DLB international workshop. Neurology 1996; 47(5):1113-24.

24. McKeith IG, Fairbairn AF, Perry RH, Thompson P, Perry EK. Neuroleptic sensitivity in patients with senile dementia of Lewy body type. British Medical Journal 1992; 305:673-8.

25. Ballard CG, Grace J, McKeith IG, Holmes C. Neuroleptic sensitivity in dementia with Lewy bodies and Alzheimer's disease. Lancet 1998; 351:1032-3.

26. The Lund and Manchester Groups. Clinical and neuropathological criteria for frontotemporal dementia. Journal of Neurology, Neurosurgery and Psychiatry 1994; 57:416-8.

27. Geschwind D, Karrim J, Nelson SF, Miller B. The apolipoprotein ε4 allele is not a significant risk factor for frontotemporal dementia. Ann Neurol 1998; 44:134-8.

28. Stewart R. Cardiovascular factors in Alzheimer's disease. Journal of Neurology, Neurosurgery and Psychiatry 1998; 65(2):143-147.

Chapter 4
Current pharmacological and psycho-social interventions

C Kelly

Cholinesterase inhibitors

Recent excitement about the cholinesterase inhibitors (CEIs), donepezil hydrochloride, and rivastigmine, followed almost three decades of treatment orientated research based upon the cholinergic deficit theory of AD (see Chapter 6). All other attempts to influence the cholinergic response in patients with AD had been disappointing. Strategies have included, precursor loading, i.e. giving choline and lecithin to increase the production of acetylcholine, enhancing the release of acetylcholine by compounds such as, phosphatidylserine, and post synaptic receptor stimulation with cholinergic agonists, e.g. pilocarpine and arecholine. The first CEI to improve cognitive function of patients with AD was the short acting physostigmine. Tacrine (1,2,3,4-tetra-hydro-9-acridinamine-monohydrochloride), because of its longer half-life, proved more useful in clinical trials. The clinical effect of the drug is modest, with 20-30% of treated patients showing improved cognitive function. In the randomised, double blind, placebo-controlled, parallel group study reported by Knapp in 1994,[29] only 279 (42%), of the 663 patients entered, completed the 30 week clinical trial. Adverse events, including elevation of liver enzymes* (LFTs), and dose related gastrointestinal symptoms, accounted for 74% of the withdrawals. Weekly monitoring of LFTs is, therefore, mandatory during the dose escalation phase. This together with the need for four times a day dosing for optimum response, has meant that Tacrine was never marketed in the UK.

Important lessons were learned by clinicians, researchers and the pharmaceutical industry from the early experience with Tacrine; all agreed that the next generation of CEIs should be:

- Less toxic

*A similar effect occurred in 29% of patients in a study of the CEI Velnacrine.

- Have a more selective CNS effect
- Have greater clinical efficacy both in cognitive and non-cognitive domains.

Donepezil hydrochloride (Aricept)

Developed by the Japanese pharmaceutical company Eisai, donepezil hydrochloride, is a piperidine-based reversible CEI that is chemically unrelated to tacrine or physostigmine. It is centrally active, possessing high selectivity for acetylcholinesterase versus butyrylcholinesterase, the latter is chiefly present outside the CNS. Its long elimination half-life of 70 hours, allows for once daily dosing - orally in the evening, with or without food - thereby improving compliance and facilitating carer supervision where necessary.

The data submitted to the regulatory bodies both in the USA and Europe, came from three randomised controlled trials involving over 1000 patients with probable AD. The key double blind 24 week study[30] was published early in 1998 and the data that follows is largely taken from this paper.

Tolerance

In clinical trials, donepezil was not hepatotoxic and no serum monitoring is, therefore, required. Pharmacokinetic studies showed no significant interaction with theophylline, cimetidine, warfarin and digoxin, but until more is known about drug interactions, patients should be monitored closely when combinations of drugs are used. Caution is required, when using neuromuscular blocking agents, e.g. succinylcholine and cholinergic agonists, in patients taking donepezil due to possible synergistic activity. Donepezil is metabolised by hepatic isoenzymes CYP2D6 and CYP3A4; inducers of these enzymes (e.g. phenytoin, carbamazepine, dexamethasone, rifampicin), and drugs which inhibit them (e.g. ketoconazole and quinidine), are likely to alter the rate of elimination of the drug.

In general, cholinomimetic drugs, including the CEIs, should be used with caution in patients with asthma or obstructive airways disease and superventricular cardiac conduction conditions and they have the potential to cause urinary retention and convulsions.

Side effects

In the phase III clinical trials[30], when the dose was increased from 5 to 10 mg after one week of treatment, gastrointestinal (GI), side effects including nausea, diarrhoea, and to a lesser extent vomiting, were more common. The total withdrawal rate at 10 mg a day dose was 16% for any adverse event. As a result, the manufacturers now suggest that the dose only be increased after one month of satisfactory response on 5 mg. Overall, both the GI and the CNS (dizziness and insomnia), side effects were mild and in most cases, transient; they occurred early and resolved within a few days of continuous treatment.

Efficacy

The primary efficacy endpoints in the phase III trials were, improvements in cognitive and global function using the ADAS-cog and CIBIC-plus (see Chapter 8). In accordance with FDA guidelines, an independent rating was made by a clinician (who remained blind to all other test results), using the Clinicians Interview Based Impression of Change with Caregiver Input (CIBIC-Plus). Four domains were looked at in this semi-structured interview including, general functioning, cognition, behaviour and activities of daily living. Using these instruments, the improvement in cognitive function in the responders was equivalent to 3-6 months delay in cognitive loss. On the 10 mg, dose, a quarter of patients showed a gain of seven or more points on the ADAS-Cog

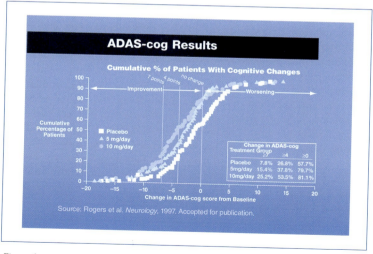

Figure 4

(*Figure 4*), equivalent to 6-12 month improvement in cognitive function. For the last six weeks of the trial all patients were given placebo. When the three groups were examined at the end of this period there were no statistical differences on any of the cognitive or global measures. This suggests that the drug effect is symptomatic only and drug withdrawal leads to the loss of any benefit. Open label extension data[31] however, have shown that donepezil produced improvements in cognition which remained superior to baseline at 38 weeks; thereafter the degree of cognitive decline was less than that reported for untreated patients. Continued administration of the drug therefore, is likely to prolong the period of cognitive gain.

Clinicians and researchers acknowledge that there is a heterogeneity of response with some patients showing a remarkable return of lost abilities, while others show either no deterioration or no measurable response. Patient genotype, vascular factors, mixed pathology, or incorrect diagnosis may all play a role but there is clearly a need to research and explain this heterogeneity of response further, in order to maximise the health gain from this and other CEIs.

Rivastigmine
Rivastigmine was licensed in the UK in June, 1998 following extensive world-wide clinical trials which included very old patients (48% >76 years), and those on multiple medications. Because of different patient populations, direct comparison cannot be made with the donepezil data. For patients receiving the higher doses of rivastigmine (6-12 mg), there was a significant improvement in cognition and activities of daily living.[32] The improvement in cognition, while of a greater numerical magnitude than that seen in the donepezil trials (4.9 versus 2.88 points on the ADAS-Cog), may not result in clinically detectable differences. The side effects are predominantly gastrointestinal during the dose titration phase. Because of a relatively short half-life, rivastigmine requires twice daily dosing. The recommended dosing regime is 1.5 mg bd for two weeks, followed by 3 mg bd for two weeks, and increasing to the highest dose of 6 mg bd if tolerated[32].

Cholinesterase inhibitors and non-cognitive symptoms
Anecdotal reports of improvements in behaviour of AD patients in clinical

trials of these drugs, have circulated for some time among investigators involved in clinical trials. There is now accumulating evidence that CEIs may indeed, improve the behavioural as well as the cognitive features of AD.

Physostigmine, a short acting CEI reduced delusional symptoms in AD patients.[33] An open label study of Tacrine[34] demonstrated significant improvement on neuropsychiatric symptoms of patients with moderate AD, and there is convincing data from the randomised double blind placebo-controlled clinical trial of Metrifonate,[35] that the drug had a significant effect on depression, apathy and hallucinations. This evidence raises a number of important issues on the use of CEIs. As carer burden is more closely related to the non-cognitive features of AD, the behavioural effects are likely to benefit carers and may explain the delay in entry to institutional care seen with Tacrine.[36] There may be, therefore, an argument for prescribing these medications for behavioural rather than cognitive-enhancing effects.

Though both donepezil and rivastigmine have been licensed for AD, from both a theoretical and a practical viewpoint they may be of equal, if not greater, benefit to patients with Dementia with Lewy bodies (DLB)[37]. The latter have been shown to have more marked cholinergic deficits in the neocortex compared with AD patients, and these deficits correlate with the presence of visual hallucinations,[38] a common presenting feature of DLB.

Making sense of the data
The effect of any therapeutic intervention is dependent on the patient sample, the circumstances of treatment and the overall management of the condition. Extrapolating meaningful data from these clinical trials to the general population of patients seen in primary and secondary care is therefore difficult. Patients in clinical trials tend to be younger and healthier with fewer complex health problems. Schneider, et al[39] from the University of Southern California School of Medicine, examined this issue further by screening their general clinic population of patients with AD, to determine the percentage that would be eligible for clinical trials.
3470 patients with possible or probable AD from nine clinics, were examined using criteria for two CEI studies. Overall, 72% of the cohort would have been excluded for either psychiatric or neurological reasons, and only 7.9% with probable AD, would have been eligible for either clinical trial. The authors concluded that these rigid entry criteria result in a skewed cohort of patients whose resemblance to the general clinic population is questionable.

There remain many unanswered questions on the contribution these drugs can make to the care of people with dementia and how best to use them. Who should receive them, when best to start, and how to rationally decide when to stop treatment, are some of the difficult decisions clinicians will increasingly face as more drugs become available (*Table 5*).

Since their introduction, public debate has concentrated on utilitarian cost effectiveness arguments that are difficult to refute as the available data does not yet exist and may not do so for some years. While it may not be appropriate to prescribe these drugs to all patients in the early stages of AD there is undoubtedly a subgroup of patients for whom such an intervention is indeed cost effective. But until substantial proof of clinical efficacy is available therapeutic nihilism will remain.

What is becomingly increasingly clear however, is that these compounds have a role to play in alleviating the clinical symptoms of AD. The choice of drug will be dictated by factors such as ease of administration (i.e. once daily dosing, no blood monitoring), least toxicity and side effects, and (all other things being equal) cost.

CHOLINESTERASE INHIBITORS				
Drug	*Reference*	*Mechanism of inhibition*	*Daily Dosing*	*Monitoring*
Tacrine	Knapp et al 1994[29]	Reversible	4	Yes
Donepezil	Rogers et al, 1996[43],96[44], 98[30]	Reversible	1	No
Rivastigmine	Anand & Enz, 1996,[45] 98[32]	Pseudo-irreversible	2	No
Metrifonate	Morris et al, 1997[46]	Pseudo-irreversible	1	
Galanthamine	Wilcock & Wilkinson, 1996[48]	Reversible	2 or 3?	

Table 5

Guidelines

Harvey in an analysis of a representative sample of guidelines produced by regional groups for the prescription of donepezil, concluded that their role appeared to be how not to prescribe the drug. In one area, the local guidelines used resulted in only two patients being prescribed the drug in six months.[40]

Shortly after the licensing of donepezil, a group of London-based old age psychiatrists suggested some criteria for the prescription and monitoring of drug treatments for AD[41] (see panel). Early in 1998, the Standing Medical Advisory Committee (SMAC), produced guidelines for the prescription of

Table 6

donepezil, unfortunately, the guidelines are specific to donepezil and cannot be generalised to all CEIs (see panel).

Who should receive treatment?

The available data suggests that this group of compounds is only of benefit to patients in the early stages of the disease. As yet, there is no convincing evidence that they are of benefit in patients with advanced disease, as they neither alter the symptoms, nor have a disease modifying effect. For optimum effect therefore, the evidence suggests that only patients with diagnosed 'probable AD', who clinically resemble the patient cohorts of clinical trials, should be prescribed these treatments. There is some evidence that apolipoprotein $\varepsilon4$ (APOE $\varepsilon4$), positive patients are less likely to respond to treatment with these drugs.[43]

Table 6 outlines issues to be considered before treatment is started. Ethical issues such as, ensuring that the patient and their carer(s) understand the diagnosis, the limitations of treatment, and that informed consent is given from the patient are of utmost importance.

Who should prescribe and monitor it?

The published guidelines suggest that specialist prescription and monitoring is required. From preceding chapters it should be clear that while the reliability of clinical diagnosis is improving, the emergence of different diagnostic categories (e.g. DLB), and the implication of vascular risk factors in AD, further shifts the assessment and early diagnosis of dementia into specialist centres.

There is an onus therefore, on health purchasers and providers to develop specialist services to meet the needs of people with dementia. This will involve not only increasing the drug budgets, but more importantly, ensuring that adequate medical, nursing, psychology and occupational therapy input is available. As experience is gained with these new drugs, treatment and management is likely to be extended into primary care, as has happened in recent years with the treatment of hypertension. Meanwhile, there is a need for increased liaison between primary and secondary care services, as traditionally, only patients with behaviour disturbance secondary to dementia have been referred for specialist assessment.

For humane and financial reasons, it is essential that drug treatment be given as part of a comprehensive package of care that must include support for the

---

MONITORING TREATMENT

Arrange early follow-up (within first month), and interview patient and carer to check compliance, tolerance and efficacy.

Document changes in the patient's medical, neurological, cognitive, behavioural, and functional status, as well as any changes in the use of medications.

Use an objective cognitive test (e.g. MMSE), to monitor efficacy.

Increase the dose according to manufacturer's recommendations and patient tolerance. Monitor caregiver's needs and level of support.

Evaluate benefit at three months using objective tests and clinician's global, as well as patient and carer, impressions.

Monitor at three monthly intervals, ensuring that the benefits of remaining on treatment outweigh the consequences of withdrawal for both the patient and carer; the lack of clinical benefit, behaviour disturbance and obvious progression of the disease, indicate when treatment should be stopped.

Table 7

unpaid family carer. Despite increased awareness of their contribution (in one small study, carers provided 79% of all care given to their behaviourally disturbed relatives with dementia), carers tend to feel ignored by health and social care professionals. Moreover, carer burnout seems inextricably linked to requests for institutional care[49], which, at present accounts for 65% of the total cost of AD in England.

How should response be assessed and judged?

The monitoring of clinical efficacy in a condition where progressive deterioration is expected, but where periodic stabilisation occurs, is problematic. As these drugs are primarily cognitive enhancers, regular monitoring of cognitive performance seems mandatory (*Table 7*). However, for carers and patients, it is the non-cognitive symptoms that cause most distress. Measures of behavioural and functional deterioration and overall clinical impression are, therefore, equally important. Where no substantial benefit has been demonstrated after three months of treatment, the drug should be stopped. Difficulties will arise where the patient has lost the ability to consent to treatment or enters institutional care; in both scenarios, most clinicians would discontinue treatment. The merits of treatment however, must be assessed on an individual basis through clinical skills and informed discussions with both the patient and carer.

Psychosocial interventions

Table 8 lists a number of recent studies that examined the effect of psychosocial interventions for patients with AD. The most interesting data have come from a study by Mary Mittelman and colleagues, based at the Ageing and Dementia Research Center of New York University. The study design was a randomised controlled intervention study in which the treatment group received: (a) two individual and four family counselling sessions; (b) a weekly support group for carers and (c) 24-hour access to trained counsellors for advice and support in times of crisis. 206 spouse caregivers of AD patients living at home, were included. All subjects were followed up twice yearly with up to eight years of follow-up. The control group was offered the standard service of the Center with intervention only as required for stabilisation or when requested. The treatment programme had the greatest effect on time to institutionalisation, with those patients in the treatment group staying an average of 329 days longer at home. The effect was greatest for those with mild or moderate AD. It is of note however, that the treatment effect was on the carer and not on the patient.

PSYCHOSOCIAL INTERVENTIONS FOR PATIENTS AND CARERS		
Author, Country, Objective design	Study Details	Results
Brodaty, & Gresham, 1989 Australia[50] Evaluation of a programme to reduce stress in carers	Carers of people with dementia in Sydney. Carers received group sessions & training in assertiveness, problem management, education & family therapy; patients given memory re-training N=36 pairs Follow-up: 12 months	Psychological morbidity was reduced in carers (P<0.05) and lower rate of patient institutionalisation
Mittelman et al, 1995, 1996 USA[48,51] Examine the effects of a support programme on depression in spouse carer-givers	Spouse care-givers living with patient with AD six sessions of counselling and carer support group Control: standard assistance given by regular staff N= 103 in both groups Follow up: 4, 8 & 12 months	Supported care-givers were less depressed than control group at eight (p<0.05) and 12 month (p<0.001), follow-up
Hinchliffe et al, 1995, UK[53] Examined the effect of individualised care packages	81 patients and 40 carers, interventions implemented over 16 weeks; control group.	Improvements demonstrated in patients and carers in Treatment group
Teri L et al 1997, USA[52] Behavioural treatment of depression in dementia patients	Two active behavioural treatments and two control groups, 72 patient-carer dyads	Significant improvements in depressive symptoms for both intervention groups

Table 8

Criticisms of the study include the absence of quality of life measures for either the patients or carers and the lack of cost-effectiveness data. While delaying entry to institutional care suggests an improved quality of life for the patient and a cost reduction, research suggests that older age, severity of dementia and being an unmarried man at the time of diagnosis, are the prime determinants of entry to institutional care. There is some concern that the delay may increase the burden and the indirect care costs to the family. Moreover, as in clinical drug trials it can be notoriously difficult to translate findings such as these to the general population of patients. Despite these drawbacks, the conclusion of the study that psychosocial interventions can contribute positively to the management of AD, now seems incontrovertible.

References:

29. Knapp MJ, Knopman DS, Solomon PR et al. A 30-week randomised controlled trial of high dose tacrine in patients with Alzheimer's disease. JAMA 1994; 271:985-991.

30. Rogers SL, Farlow MR, Doody RS, et al. A 24-week double blind placebo-controlled trial of donepezil in patients with Alzheimer's disease. Neurology 1998; 50:136-145.

31. Rogers SL, Friedhoff LT. Long-term efficacy and safety of donepezil in the treatment of Alzheimer's disease: an interim analysis of the results of a US multicentre open label extension study. European Neuropsychopharmacology 1998; 8:67-75.

32. Corey-Bloom J, Anand R and Veach J. A randomised trial evaluating the efficacy and safety of ENA 713 (rivastigmine tartrate), a new acetyl cholinesterase inhibitor, in patients with mild to moderately severe Alzheimer's disease. International Journal of Geriatric Psychopharmacology 1998; 1:55-65.

33. Cummings JL, Gorman DG, Shapira J. Physostigmine ameliorates the delusions of Alzheimer's disease. Biol Psychiatry1993; 33:536-541.

34. Kaufer D, Cummings JL, Chrstine D. Differential neuropsychiatric response to tacrine in Alzheimer's disease: relationship to dementia severity. Journal of Neuropsychiatry and Clinical Neurosciences 1998; 10:55-63.

35. Morris J, Cyrus P, Orazem J, Mas J, Bieber F, Gulanski B. Effects of metrifonate on the cognitive, global, and behavioral function of Alzheimer's disease patients: results of a randomised, double blind, placebo-controlled study. Neurology 1997; 48:1730 Abstract.

36. Knopman D, Schneider L, Davis K et al. Long term tacrine treatment: effects on nursing home placement and mortality. Neurology 1996; 47:166-7.

37. Langlais PJ, Thal LJ, Hansen L, et al. Neurotransmitters in basal ganglia and cortex of Alzheimer's disease with and without Lewy bodies. Neurology 1993; 43:1927-1934.

38. Perry EK, Marshall E, Kerwin JM et al. Evidence of a monaminergic:cholinergic imbalance related to visual hallucinations in Lewy body dementia. J Neurochem 1990; 55:1454-1456.

39. Schneider LS, Olin JT, Lyness SA, Chui HC. Eligibility of Alzheimer's disease clinic patients for clinical trials. J Am Geriatr Soc 1997; 45:923-928.

40. Harvey RJ. The use of guidelines for the prescription of cholinergic inhibitors. International J Geriatric Psychiatry 1998; in press.

41. Lovestone S, Graham N, Howard R, Harvey R, Kelly C et al. Guidelines on drug treatments for Alzheimer's disease. Lancet 1997; 350:232-3.

42. SMAC Guidance to clinicians on the use of donepezil for Alzheimer's disease. NHS Executive 1998.

43. Selkoe DJ. Alzheimer's disease: genotypes, phenotypes and treatments. Science 1997; 275:630-1.

44. Rogers SL, Doody R, Mohs R et al. E2020 produces both clinical global and cognitive test improvement in patients with mild to moderately severe Alzheimer's disease: results of a 30-week Phase III trial [abstract]. Neurology 1996; 46 (suppl):A217.

45. Rogers SL, Friedhoff LT, and the donepezil study group. The efficacy and safety of donepezil in patients with Alzheimer's disease: results of a US multicentre, randomised, double blind, placebo-controlled trial. Dementia 1996; 7:293-303.

46. Anand R, Gharabawi G Enz A. Efficacy and safety results of the early Phase III studies with Exelon (ENA-713) in Alzheimer's disease: an overview. J Drug Dev Clin Pract 1996; 8:109-116.

47. Morris JC, Cyrus PA, Orazem J et al. Metrifonate benefits cognitive, behavioural and global function in patients with Alzheimer's disease. Neurology; 50:1222-1230.

48. Wilcock G, Wilkinson D. Galanthamine hydrobromide: interim results of a group comparative, placebo controlled study of efficacy and safety in patients with a diagnosis of senile dementia of the Alzheimer's type. Neurobiology of Aging 1996; 17(suppl4S):S144.

49. Mittelman MS, Ferris SH, Shulman E, Steinberg G, Levin B. A family intervention study to delay nursing home placement of patients with Alzheimer's disease. JAMA 1996; 276:1725-1731.

50. Brodaty H, Gresham M. Effects of a training programme to reduce stress in carers of patients with dementia. BMJ 1989; 299:1375-1379.

51. Mittelman MS, Ferris SH, Shulman E, et al. A comprehensive support programme: effect on depression in spouse caregivers of AD patients. Gerontologist 1995; 35:792-802.

52. Teri Linda, Behavioural treatment of depression in dementia patients: a controlled clinical trial. Journal of Gerontology, Series B. Psychological Sciences & Social Sciences. Vol 52b(4). July 1997; p159-166.

53. Hinchliffe AC, Hyman IL, Blizard, B, Livingston G. Behavioural complications of dementia. International Journal of Geriatric Psychiatry, Vol 10 (10), October 1995; p839-847.

Chapter 5

Treatment in dementia: ethical and legal issues[54]

Martin J Vernon

Introduction

Dementia is a progressive disease process which erodes the decision making capacity of adults over a period of months or years. During that time, the need for healthcare interventions may increase, while often the benefit-to-risk ratio of treatment decreases. Some of the most important healthcare decisions of an individual's life may need to be taken following the onset of dementia, at a time when they are cognitively least able to participate in the decision making process.

The nature of dementia creates huge scope for overriding treatment choices, particularly where capacity to make decisions has been only partly eroded. A patient pulling away from a needle prick may have decided to refuse treatment, or may be displaying reflexive behaviour consequent upon impaired 'executive function'.[55] Alternatively, a patient may appear to agree to treatment, unable to communicate their refusal or having failed to understand relevant information. Such difficulties may prompt the unsound conclusion that the patient cannot decide, and that the decision should be taken on their behalf.

English Consent Law

English law upholds the right of adults to accept or refuse medical treatment without having to justify their decision (see page 41). Driven by the ethical principle of respect for autonomy, the law protects individuals from unwanted interference, and there is little legal or ethical justification for overriding a patient's competently made treatment decision, even when this causes them harm. The House of Lords has clearly stated the consequences for a doctor who attempts to proceed with treatment in the absence of his patient's consent:

A doctor who operates without the consent of his patient is, save in the cases of emergency or mental disability, guilty of the civil wrong of trespass to the person; he is also guilty of the criminal offence of assault.[56]

For patients who are incompetent, the situation is less clear. No one else can provide a legally valid consent for adults who lack competence,[57,58] and there is surprisingly little legal or ethical guidance available to professionals faced with treating an incompetent patient. As a result, individuals may lose their right to decide about treatment, becoming the subjects of care planning over which they have little or no control.

Legal justification for treatment of incompetent adults is derived from the principle of necessity, contingent upon treatment being in the patient's *best interests*.[59] Establishing best interests involves weighing the interests a patient may have in receiving treatment against not receiving it. Doctors should act in accordance with a responsible body of medical opinion when weighing interests,[59, 61] but this may cause problems when an incompetent patient refuses treatment. Doctors may proceed lawfully if a responsible body of professional opinion concludes that treatment is in the patient's best interests, but the incompetent adult has no legal right of refusal, even when supported by a second body of opinion which holds that such treatment is not in their best interests.[61]

Dementia, autonomy and personhood
By granting an individual the legal right to self-determination, it is assumed that they are capable of self-governance, and that within the individual resides a self in need of governance. A demented patient's right to decide about medical treatment is thus, in part, contingent upon the presence of both *autonomy* (to which the notion of self-governance is central)[62,63], and *personhood*.

i) Does the onset of dementia destroy autonomy?
The concept of autonomy is linked to that of freedom.[66] There are few situations where an individual is truly free from all interference, and arguably, patients with limited autonomy through illness are no different from other 'fully' autonomous individuals.[65] The spectrum of cognitive impairments which supervene in dementia may restrict a patient's freedom, but such restriction need only *limit* their autonomy rather than destroy it altogether.

An autonomous individual must be able and free to choose between desires if they are to have any control over their life. Consider a patient whose swallowing is impaired, for which problem her doctor has decided to insert a nasogastric feeding tube. Her desires to stop feeling hungry and to stop feeling the

LEGAL FRAMEWORK FOR TREATING PATIENTS WITH DEMENTIA

Is the patient competent?

Can patient understand and retain information?
Can patient weigh information to arrive at a choice?

Yes

No

Does statue permit overriding?
(eg Mental Health Act 1983, s63)

**Is treatment necessary
and in patient's best interests?**

Yes

No

Yes

No

If proposed treatment
falls within terms of
statute, it may be
legal to proceed
without consent

Treatment may
proceed even in face
of patient's refusal

Patient's decision
(acceptance or refusal)
must be respected

No common law
justification for
proceedings

discomfort of the tube are in conflict. If she wants the desire to stop feeling hungry to be effective, she will continue with the tube despite discomfort. Alternatively, she may want the desire not to be in discomfort to be effective, and she will pull the tube out. It is the ability to choose between and make effective particular desires which indicates that the patient is acting autonomously.[66]

If the patient has dementia, there are two ways in which her autonomy may be challenged. Firstly, the disease may prevent the patient from rendering effective her desires. For example, loss of purposeful movement may prevent her from pulling out the tube, or perceptual failure may prevent satiety. Second, loss of executive function may prevent her from choosing between desires, so that whichever desire is the stronger (lack of hunger or lack of discomfort), becomes effective.

There are problems with this approach. It may be tempting to assume that a patient who repeatedly pulls out a feeding tube is responding to the strong desire to be comfortable and therefore not autonomous. However, there is nothing in her actions to distinguish whether or not she is making an autonomous choice. Failure to make effective a particular desire may be because the patient favours a different desire, or it may be because her impairments prevent her from doing so.

Nevertheless, the presence or absence of executive function is a useful clinical marker of whether the patient is capable of choosing between desires and therefore of behaving autonomously. An individual unable to organise, plan and initiate action will act reflexively, losing control over their desires, and losing their autonomy for action. On the other hand impairments which disrupt perception or communication will make assessment of autonomy difficult, but do not necessarily abolish autonomy.

ii) Does the onset of dementia destroy personhood?
The characteristics which define a person include rationality and awareness of self.[67] Arguably, dementia poses the greatest threat to personhood via its effects on rationality. The characteristics of rational behaviour, namely choice, human purpose, awareness of action and intention, will be less in evidence when an individual can no longer recall past events, communicate with others, execute purposeful movement, perceive sensory phenomena or modulate reflexive behaviour.[68] However, personhood and irrationality may

not be mutually exclusive; most of us are aware of the dangers of smoking, drinking too much alcohol or driving too fast, and yet we retain personhood, notwithstanding such irrational behaviour. While the onset of dementia may threaten an individual's rationality, their irrational behaviour may not, of necessity, indicate a loss of personhood.

Self-awareness in dementia poses less difficulty. One view of self is that of a being which 'is able to entertain first person thoughts'.[69] The ability to ascribe first person thoughts to a being may be sufficient for the recognition of self-awareness in an individual.[69] Take the example of a patient with dementia who evokes the comment, 'she is pleased with herself today', from her relatives. Such an ascribed thought indicates that her relatives at least regard her as self aware. Except in the most impaired patient, it is hard to imagine a situation where this criterion would not be met; loss of speech or social function may impede the communication of first person thoughts, but it is not until the advanced stages of dementia that ascribable thoughts lose their meaning.

It is less clear whether the changes which occur in thoughts and experiences as a result of dementia lead to awareness of a *different* self from that which existed prior to the onset of disease. This is illustrated by the case of a man who cannot remember past events from his life, recognise his family, or even his own image in a mirror. His self-awareness is evidenced by statements such as, 'I want to eat' or 'I am in pain', but since he cannot recognise any characteristics of his prior existence, is the self of which he is now aware a different self? Indeed, is he a different *person* altogether?

Legal basis of treatment in dementia
So long as they remain competent, patients with dementia have the same, almost unqualified legal right to decide about their treatment as all other adults. The key to this legal right is competence.

i) legal meaning of capacity
Competence or *capacity* [70] may be viewed from two legal perspectives, namely *status* and *functional ability* to decide.

a) status approach
With this approach incapacity is determined by characteristics which describe

a group of individuals, for example age under sixteen or the presence of mental illness. This is problematic because of its poor specificity; some individuals within the defined group may actually have capacity. The courts have, therefore, taken the view that a status approach to capacity is not workable; an individual's capacity cannot be decided on the basis of their intelligence, education or mental health.[58,71,72] The presence of mental illness, as defined in the Mental Health Act 1983, does not equate with incapacity, and doctors treating patients under the terms of the Act are not absolved from determining their patient's capacity to decide.[73] A dementia sufferer cannot be deemed legally incompetent purely on the grounds of their mental health status, even when their disorder is sufficiently severe to warrant detention under the 1983 Act.

b) Functional approach

The law takes a functional view of capacity broadly based on *understanding*. Although there are successively more demanding standards against which a patient may be tested, the Courts have generally supported the lowest standard which tests *ability* to understand. A competent patient will therefore, be able to understand in *broad terms* what a proposed treatment involves. In addition, determination of understanding should be contemporaneous with the planned treatment: capacity is only absent for as long as the ability to understand is impaired. For a dementing patient whose cognition varies day by day, it is thus important to establish their capacity *at the time* of the proposed treatment.

ii) Presumption and continuance

The law presumes all adults to have capacity until proven otherwise. *Presumption* removes the burden from a patient to prove their capacity and it is for others to provide evidence that the patient lacks capacity. Failure to do so leaves intact the patient's capacity and, therefore, their right to choose. Having proven incapacity however, proof to the contrary will be required before a patient is deemed competent again. This principle of *continuance* is troublesome when a patient's mental function varies over time. Once a dementing patient is found to be incompetent, continuance may mitigate against the restoration of capacity despite periods of lucidity.

iii) Establishing capacity

The courts have issued guidance on the criteria which should be applied by professionals when establishing capacity. In the case of *Re C*, which concerned a man with schizophrenia refusing surgical removal of a gangrenous leg, the judge formulated a legal test, failure of which would constitute sufficient evidence to rebut the presumption of capacity.[71] A patient therefore, has capacity if he is able to:

- understand and retain information
- believe it
- weigh it in the balance to arrive at a choice.

In a more recent case[74] the Court of Appeal modified this test by placing less importance on belief, which arguably renders patients incompetent simply because they choose not to believe their doctor. It is important to notice that this *legal* test of capacity does not equate with *clinical* tests of cognitive function; a poor performance in the latter does not connote legal incapacity. Clinical tests of cognition must not be substituted for legal tests of capacity.

Legal reform

In an overview of consent law in 1991, the Law Commission recognised legal difficulties at the capacity/incapacity interface, and in particular the vulnerability of incapacitated adults in respect of health care decision making.[75] It acknowledged tensions between professional duties to help patients, and public interests in protecting vulnerable individuals from well-intentioned but inappropriate treatment or, conversely, deprivation of health care through rationing.[76] In proposing new legislation to govern decision making for incapacitated adults, the legal approach to incapacity was seen as pivotal. Broadly, two approaches are open to the government:

a) to elevate the legal threshold for incapacity
b) to improve the legal rules protecting incapacitated adults.

The Commission in general favours approach a). It recommends a legal presumption against incapacity, and the presence of 'mental disability',[77] and/or inability to communicate as minimum requirements for incapacity. A test of incapacity has been synthesised, aimed at enabling and empowering individuals on the threshold of incapacity. An individual thus lacks capacity by *reason of mental disability* if they are unable to:

- understand or retain relevant information, and
- make a decision based on relevant information.

Information must be presented in broad terms and simple language, and include reasonably foreseeable consequences. Such an approach seeks to 'import a patient's right to information'[78] into the test for capacity, but the obvious problem is the degree of control an information provider may have over a patient's capacity.

This test gives clarity to the definition of legal incapacity, but concerns remain at both the extent to which such a formulation truly enables and empowers patients at the threshold of incapacity, and the application of such proposals in practice. While elevating the threshold for incapacity, the Commission has left professionals with opportunities to arbitrate decisions about their patients' capacity. In particular, the quality of information (rather than the language used to communicate it), provided to the patient may fall under the direct control of professionals whose task it is to decide if capacity is present or absent. The Commission acknowledges that doctors presently may vary the criteria by which capacity is judged in order to secure the outcome they desire, and to an extent such opportunities would persist should the proposals become law.

Conclusion

Adults with dementia have a legal right to decide about treatment based on the principle of respect for autonomy. For those without capacity the law offers paternalistic solutions to treatment decisions, over which the patient has little control. While dementia does not render patients legally incompetent, it is difficult to apply existing legal standards to individuals with impaired powers of communication, perception or execution. In addition, while presumption of capacity protects patients with declining cognition, the principle of continuance undermines those whose cognition varies. This may generate false assumptions about capacity and permit professionals to override their patient's valid treatment decisions.

The Law Commission has suggested reforms that seek to empower individuals with cognitive impairment, but the law is likely to remain entrenched with the principle of respect for autonomy. This approach ensures that a patient's right to decide about treatment is contingent upon their being autonomous. It does not necessarily protect the rights of those whose autonomy is impaired. For this reason, patients with dementia may be served better by a legal framework based on promotion of benefit or avoidance of harm.

These issues will assume greater importance as new and expensive treatments for dementia become available. Participation in a clinical trial is limited by a patient's capacity to consent. In consequence the evaluation of novel treatments is confined to patients with early disease, and their efficacy in advanced dementia remains unknown. Those with advanced disease may be denied potentially beneficial treatment, while the absence of trial data will continue to justify the rationing of health resources among patients with dementia. Changes to the legal frameworks and professional values governing consent to treatment may have far-reaching consequences.

Key points

- Adults have a legal right to accept or refuse medical treatment without having to justify their decision

- No one else can provide a legally valid consent for adults who lack capacity

- Legal justification for treatment of incompetents is derived from the principle of necessity, decided by weighing best interests

- The law presumes adults to have capacity, but once found to be incompetent, continuance may mitigate against restoration of capacity despite periods of lucidity

- The Law Commission has proposed legal reform which protects vulnerable adults by raising the legal threshold for incapacity

- A patient has legal capacity if he is able to understand and retain information, and weigh it in the balance to arrive at a choice

- Capacity to decide about treatment is contingent upon autonomy and personhood, which may be eroded by dementia

- Executive function is a clinical marker of a patient's capability of behaving autonomously

- Dementia threatens personhood via its effects on rationality, but irrational behaviour does not necessarily indicate incapacity.

Legal footnotes

54. Adapted from: *Consent to treatment in dementia: right or privilege?* Vernon MJ. Dissertation submitted for the degree of Master of Arts in Medical Ethics and Law, King's College London, 1998.

55. *Sidaway v Bethlem Royal Hospital Governors* [1985] 1 All ER 643.

56. *T v T* [1988] Fam 52.

57. *Re T (adult: refusal of medical treatment)* [1992] 4 All ER 649.

58. *Re F* [1989] 2 All ER 545.

59. *Bolam v Friern Hospital Management Committee [1957] 2 All ER118.*

60. Jones MA, Keywood K. *Assessing the patient's competence to consent to medical treatment.* [1996] 2 Med Law Int 107.

61. *Principles of Biomedical Ethics (4th Edition).* Beauchamp TL, Childress JF (1994): Oxford, Oxford University Press.

62. *The Value of Life,* Harris J (1985): London, Routledge.

63. *Four Essays on Liberty,* Berlin I (1969); Oxford, Oxford University Press.

64. *Paternalism and partial autonomy.* O'Neill O (1984): Journal of Medical Ethics; 10: 173-178.

65. For a full philosophical discussion of this approach, see *Freedom of will and the concept of a person.* Frankhurt HG (1971): Journal of Philosophy 68, pp5-20.

66. *Rethinking life and death.* Singer P (1995): Oxford, Oxford University Press.

67. See *Diagnostic and Statistical Manual of Mental Disorders (4th Edition)* (DSM-IV) American Psychiatric Association (1994): Washington DC, APA.

68. *The Oxford Companion to Philosophy.* Honderich T (ed) (1995): Oxford, Oxford University Press pp 816-817.

69. The terms competence and capacity are used here interchangeably.

70. *Re C (refusal of medical treatment),* [1994] 1 FLR 31.

71. *St George's Healthcare NHS Trust v S,* [1998] TLR 299.

72. Under s63 of the 1983 Act, patients liable to be detained may be treated for the relevant mental disorder without their consent, subject to certain exceptions (e.g. psychosurgery, hormonal implantation, electro-convulsive therapy, see s57 and s58). However in a number of celebrated court decisions (e.g. *B v Croydon Health Authority* [1995] 1 All ER 693) the meaning of 'treatment for the disorder' has been extended to include 'ancillary treatment' such as tube feeding and nursing care.

73. *Re MB* [1997] 8 Med L R 217.

74. Mentally Incapacitated Adults and Decision-Making: An overview (1991), Consultation Paper No. 119.

75. Mentally Incapacitated Adults and Decision-Making: Medical Treatment and Research (1993), Consultation Paper No. 129.

76. The Commission sets out an interesting discussion on the merits of using the term 'mental disability' rather than 'disorder' as defined in the Mental Health Act 1983. Although the latter is seen as both restrictive and stigmatising, having been used largely in the sphere of psychiatric disease, the arguments more properly give voice to wider policy concerns. Increasingly, society has shifted focus from an individual's physical or mental impairment to the impact of that impairment on their function and role. It has been recognised that disease does not equate with disability, and new legislation must take account of this by favouring a subjective, functional approach centred on the individual's response to their impairment. Such an approach would be particularly useful in dementia, where compensatory mechanisms may preserve function in a patient whose objective cognition is severely impaired.

77. *Statutory Authority to Treat, Relatives and Treatment Proxies* (1994) 2 Med L Rev 30.

78. Who Decides? Making Decisions on Behalf of Mentally Incapacitated Adults. (1997) Lord Chancellor's Department at 11 to 13.

PART 2 - THEORY

Chapter 6

Aetiology of Alzheimer's Disease

F Burnett

NEUROPATHOLOGY

The clinical syndrome of AD results from molecular changes and cellular dysfunction in the brain. Recent advances in the understanding of this process have created opportunities for therapeutic interventions at earlier stages of the disease.

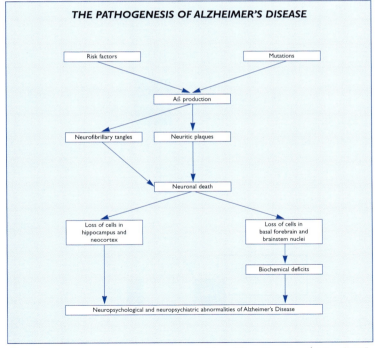

Figure 5   *Adapted from Cummings & Mega (1996).*

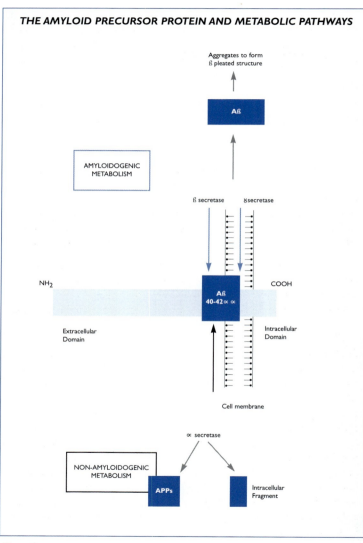

Figure 6

ß-amyloid

Deposition of ß-amyloid (Aß) in the brain is central to the pathogenesis of AD. Aß is a 40-42 amino acid peptide which is derived from the large transmembranous amyloid precursor protein (APP). There are two main routes of APP metabolism, both of which occur in health (*Figure 6*). Increased metabolism by the amyloidogenic pathway is probably harmful. Approximately 10% of Aß produced is the relatively insoluble Aß42, (43) which preferentially aggregates in a ß-pleated configuration. In its insoluble aggregated form, Aß is toxic to neurones and causes apoptotic cell death in vitro.

The regulation of APP metabolism is incompletely understood. Expression of APP appears to be increased by neuronal injury or oxidative/ischaemic stress, and by trisomy of the APP gene on chromosome 21. Certain genetic mutations seem to promote amyloidogenic metabolism, as do cytotoxic events causing increased intracellular calcium. The non-amyloidogenic pathway may be triggered by neuronal stimulation by acetyl choline and other neurotransmitters.[79]

The distinctive histopathological features of AD are senile plaques and neurofibrillary tangles in the neocortex and hippocampus. Other neuropathological characteristics include granulovacuolar degeneration, Hirano bodies, and Aß deposition in the walls of small cortical blood vessels.

Senile plaques

Senile plaques are extracellular structures consisting of a core of Aß fibrils surrounded by dystrophic neurites, astrocytes and microglia. The plaques also contain proteins that provide clues about the pathophysiology of AD including apolipoproteins and inflammatory proteins such as α-1-antichymotrypsin, protein kinase C and complement. Mature plaques appear to develop from diffuse forms which are present in the brains of non-demented older people. Normal neurites in the vicinity of diffuse plaques may be damaged by the toxic effects of unaggregated Aß or other factors. The density of senile plaques does not correlate with the severity of cognitive impairment, however the diagnosis of AD relies upon exceeding the normal age specific density of senile plaques. Patients with mild AD will already have appreciable numbers of plaques in the neocortex, and plaques may be present for ten years before AD is clinically detectable.[79, 80]

Neurofibrillary tangles

NFTs are intraneuronal structures consisting of paired helical filaments containing the microtubule-associated protein, tau. The participation of tau in the structure of the neuronal cytoskeleton is dependent on the degree of phosphorylation which is controlled by protein kinases and phosphatases. In an abnormally hyperphosphorylated state, tau forms paired helical filaments, disrupts microtubule formation and leads to cell death. High intracellular calcium leads to NFT formation, and loss of calcium homeostasis may be the common factor shared by plaques and tangles.[81] In AD the density of NFT in the neocortex correlates with the severity of dementia, however age related deposits are present in the hippocampus and inferior temporal cortex in people without dementia. NFTs accumulate in response to a variety of degenerative, toxic and traumatic insults to the brain.

Neuronal damage

Normal aging is associated with a reduction in brain weight beginning in the 5th or 6th decade in women and a decade later in men. In AD there is progressive neuronal shrinkage and death affecting multiple brain areas including the hippocampus, brain stem, basal forebrain, frontal and temporoparietal areas of the neocortex. Typically this leads to diffuse cortical atrophy and dilatation of the ventricles in the late stages.

Multiple factors may participate in AD related neuronal damage. There is evidence that free radicals may be involved in promoting Aß aggregation because antioxidants inhibit Aß fibril formation. Aß fibrils may enhance free

---

CAUSES OF NEURONAL DAMAGE IN ALZHEIMER'S DISEASE

Direct toxic effects of beta amyloid

Free radicals promote Aß aggregation

Neurofibrillary tangles disrupt microtubule formation

Altered cell membrane function causes Ca^{2+} influx (excitotoxicity)

Immune mechanisms: activation of complement pathways causes cell lysis

? Expression of Par-4 protein promotes apoptosis

Table 9

radical formation which damage cell membranes leading to altered calcium homeostasis.[80] Recent research has identified a 15-20 fold increase in the concentration of the prostate apoptosis response-4 (Par-4) protein and its mRNA in post mortem hippocampal tissue from subjects with AD. This protein appears to be a marker of neuronal apoptosis and is predominantly expressed in cells with accumulations of NFT. Hippocampal cells exposed in vitro to Aß also show marked induction of Par-4. The significance of these findings is unclear, however it is suggested that Par-4 develops after exposure to the neuropathological markers of AD.[82] Blockade of Par-4 expression or function may inhibit neuronal apoptosis and could lead to new therapeutic interventions.

Increased intracellular calcium causes cell death by a process called excitotoxicity. The glial response to neuronal injury involves activation of the complement pathway and terminates in the membrane attack complex which causes cell lysis. An enhanced immune response in AD produces chronic inflammation, and anti-inflammatory drugs may limit the neuronal injury caused by this process.

NEUROTRANSMITTERS
Cell death in the forebrain and brain stem nuclei leads to deficits in the synthesis of neurotransmitters in AD, and altered receptor function may contribute to the neuropathological process.

The Cholinergic System
The cholinergic system is believed to be involved in the functions of memory and learning. Cholinergic innervation of the neocortex and hippocampus originates from the nucleus basilis of Meynert (nbM) in the basal forebrain. The nbM manufactures choline acetyl transferase (CAT) which synthesises acetyl choline and is a pre-synaptic cholinergic marker. Neuronal loss in the nbM and progressive loss of CAT activity correlate with senile plaque formation and dementia severity. Loss of cholinergic cortical neurones tends to be greatest in the temporal cortex and amygdala (up to 85%). Several receptor studies have demonstrated reduction in the density of nicotinic receptors and possible functional alterations of muscarinic receptors.

Underactivity of cholinergic pathways may promote amyloidogenic APP metabolism and senile plaque formation. The cholinergic deficit in AD provides the rationale for cholinomimetic therapy. Cholinesterase inhibitors reduce the breakdown of acetyl choline and have been shown to be modestly effective in improving the cognitive deficits in AD (see Chapter 4).

CHOLINERGIC DEFICITS IN ALZHEIMER'S DISEASE

Atrophy of cells in the Nucleus Basilis of Meynert

Loss of cholinergic cortical neurones
    ↓ choline acetyl transferase synthesis
    ↓ acetyl choline synthesis
    ↓ density of nicotinic receptors

? functional change of muscarinic receptors

Cholinergic underactivity may promote amyloidogenic metabolism and senile plaque formation

---

Table 10

The Serotonergic System

Evidence from animal and human studies suggest that serotonin (5-HT) is involved in the functions of mood, aggression, feeding and sleep. Dysregulation of 5-HT is central to the pathogenesis of depression, and is linked to impulsivity and suicidal behaviour. It may also play a role in memory and learning through its close links to the cholinergic system.

The raphe nucleus which is an area of high serotonergic neuronal density, is a preferential site for NFT formation and neuronal loss in AD. Reduced 5-HT content has been demonstrated throughout the neocortex, with an increased 5-HIAA/5-HT ratio reflecting turnover. Significant reductions in presynaptic 5-HT re-uptake sites ($5-HT_2$ receptors) have been demonstrated. These receptors are localised on glutaminergic pyramidal neurons and on cholinergic nerve terminals and may reflect loss of these cells in AD. Patients assessed during life as having prominent behavioural symptoms show more marked loss of serotonergic uptake sites in the neocortex at post mortem. Drugs which enhance serotonergic neurotransmission such as SSRIs and trazodone may improve mood and behavioral symptoms, however there is little evidence that they have an effect on cognitive function.

Noradrenaline (NA)

Noradrenaline levels have been shown to be depleted in the cortex, particularly in temporal and parietal areas in several post mortem studies of AD. A corresponding loss of noradrenergic neurones and NFT deposition have been documented in the locus coeruleus from where the hippocampus and neocortex receive their noradrenergic innervation. Reduction in binding of the presynaptic $\alpha 2$ noradrenergic autoreceptor in AD probably reflects loss of noradrenergic afferents. It has been suggested that NA is important in preventing distraction by irrelevant stimuli. So far, no study of noradrenergic agents have reported any improvement of cognitive function in AD.

Dopamine

The number of dopaminergic neurones declines with age in normal humans. The majority of dopaminergic neurones in the brain originate in the substantia nigra and in the ventral tegmental area. AD appears to be associated with a modest degree of cell loss in these brain areas. Deficits in indices of dopaminergic function are considerably greater when Lewy bodies

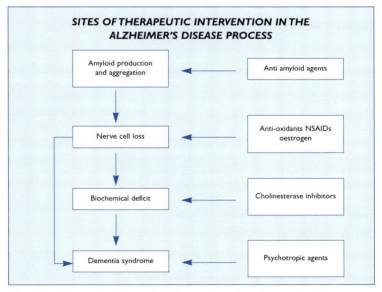

Figure 7. Adapted from J. Cummings. Presentation at 151st APA Meeting, Toronto, 998.

are present in the neocortex and substantia nigra. Dementia of Lewy body type is also associated with relatively greater cholinergic deficits.

Glutamate

Glutamate is an excitatory neurotransmitter that is involved in the major input and output pathways from the hippocampus. Several studies have indicated that the severity of cognitive deficit in AD correlates with the degeneration of pyramidal neurones in the parietotemporal cortex in which glutamate is the major neurotransmitter. There is also acceleration of the age related decrease in density of the N-methyl-D-aspartate (NMDA) receptor in the hippocampus and neo-cortex. Excessive stimulation of glutamate receptors causes calcium influx into neurons resulting in cell damage or death (excitotoxicity), which may play a role in neuronal degeneration in AD.

Reduced activity of glutaminergic neurones has been implicated in the mechanisms leading to hyperphosphorylation of tau and NFT formation. Glutamate stimulation of rat cortical neurons reduces the generation of paired helical filament -like tau[83].

GENETICS

Age at onset of dementia is important in determining the influence of genetic factors in cases of AD. In the 5% of affected individuals who become symptomatic before the age of 65, the disease appears to be linked to highly penetrant autosomal dominant genetic lesions. Typically half of the offspring of such people will be affected. To date, causative mutations have been identified on chromosomes 21, 14 and 1, however only 30-50% of all known pedigrees with early-onset familial AD can be linked to any of the known mutations. Overall, the APOE genotype is the single most common genetic determinant of susceptibility to AD and may account for up to 50% of the risk for developing late onset familial and sporadic AD[84]. The discovery of further genetic vulnerability factors is anticipated.

Early Onset Familial Alzheimer's Disease

The Amyloid Precursor Gene

Several mutations on the gene for the APP on chromosome 21 have been linked to early onset familial AD. These mutations lie outside the ß amyloid protein domain on APP, and may alter proteolytic processing causing production of longer fragments of Aß which are more likely to aggregate. This hypothesis is supported by studies of transgenic mice overexpressing mutant human APP genes. The animals produce increased amounts of Aß42, (43), deposit human Aß in the brain with increasing age and display age related memory deficits[85]. Down's syndrome with three copies of the APP gene on chromosome 21 is invariably associated with AD pathology in mid-life.

CHROMOSOMES	GENES	EFFECTS OF THE MUTATION
Chromosome 21	Amyloid Precursor Protein	Promotes amyloidogenic metabolism and Aß deposition
Chromosome 14	Presenilin-1 protein	Promotes Aß deposition
Chromosome 1	Presenilin - 2 protein	Promotes Aß deposition
Chromosome 19	APOE genotype	Facilitates Aß deposition May affect NFT formation Affects vulnerability to risk

Table 11

The Presenilin Genes
Genetic linkage analysis led to the identification of a second familial AD locus on chromosome 14 subsequently named the presenilin-1 gene (PS-1). Mutations of the PS-1 gene probably account for the majority cases of early onset familial AD.

Sequences homologous to the PS-1 gene were identified on chromosome 1 indicating the existence of a second presenilin gene (PS-2). Genetic linkage between familial AD and DNA markers on chromosome 1 were detected in the Volga German pedigree and in an Italian pedigree. Families with PS-2 mutations show a range of age of onset (44-88 years) and incomplete penetrance. Mutations of this gene are probably a rare cause of AD.

The structure of presenilins suggests a role in cell membrane function. Studies of homologous protein sequences from the nematode Caenorhabditis elegans suggest that they may have a role in determining cell fate during development. Fibroblasts from affected individuals with PS mutations secrete relatively increased proportions of fibrillogenic Aß42, (43) compared with unaffected family members[86], and transgenic mice carrying the mutant PS-1 gene have twice as much Aß42, (43) in the brain compared with normal mice.

Late Onset Alzheimer's Disease

The Apolipoprotein E (APOE)Gene

APOE is involved in lipid transport and metabolism. The APOE gene is located on chromosome 19, and exists in three allelic forms: APOE ε2, ε3, and ε4. The APOE ε4 allele shows a dose dependent increase in the risk of developing AD, apparently mediated through a decrease in the age of onset of the disease. The risk of developing AD is increased three fold for heterozygotes carrying the ε4 allele, and by eight fold for homozygotes.[84] Despite this some APOE ε4 carriers remain cognitively intact throughout their lifetime. The association with the genotype occurs sporadically, but is more robust in familial forms .

The biological basis for the association between the ε4 allele and AD is unclear. Evidence suggests that APOE genotype may interact with environmental risk factors such as head injury to increase the likelihood of AD developing.[97] APOE is found in senile plaques, and the ε4 allele may facilitate aggregation of Aß. Deposition of Aß appears to be correlated with the number of ε4 alleles, and the APOE ε2 genotype may be associated with a reduced risk of Aß deposition. APOE binds to tau and the allelic form may influence NFT formation.

Pathological data indicates that APOE ε4 alleles show an inverse relationship with residual brain choline acetyltransferase activity and nicotinic receptor density.[87] This suggests that individuals with APOE ε4 alleles may respond less well to cholinomimetic therapies because they have less residual cholinergic innervation.

The α 2 macroglobulin gene

Very recent reports have implicated a common variant of the α2 macroglobulin

gene in the aetiology of late onset familial AD[88] . This variant may be
implicated in the clearance of Aß from the synaptic cleft. It is present in 20%
of the population and the level of risk may be the same as that conferred by
APOE ε4 genotype, however it remains to be established whether the
pedigree studies can be applied to the general population.

RISK FACTOR	RELATIVE RISK (95 % CI)
Family history of dementia	3.5 (2.6-4.6)
Family history of Down's syndrome	2.7 (1.2-5.7)
Hypothyroidism	2.3 (1.0-5.4)
Epilepsy	1.6 (0.7-3.5)
Head trauma	1.8 (1.3-2.7)
Depression	1.8 (1.2-2.9)
Smoking	0.8 (0.6-1.0)

Adapted from van Duijn, C.M., Hofman, A.(1992) Risk factors for Alzheimer's disease: the EURODEM
collaborative re-analysis of case-control studies. Neuroepidemiology; 11(suppl 1): 106-113

Table 12

Chromosome 12

A recent study involving a complete genomic screen of 16 families affected by
late onset AD identified a strong and consistent region of interest on
chromosome 12, and other susceptibility markers on chromosomes 4, 6, and
20.[89] These findings have yet to be replicated, however if candidate genes are
identified these are likely to provide further clues about the pathophysiology
of AD.

RISK FACTORS

No specific cause is found in most patients with AD, however a variety of risk
factors have been identified from epidemiological studies. A role for
environmental factors is supported by studies that demonstrate a 40%
concordance rate for monozygotic twins and a variation in age of onset in
concordant pairs.

Demographic factors

The risk of developing dementia doubles every five years after the age of 65. With increasing age the rate of neuronal death increases, there has been more time for the effects genes to be expressed and for exposure to toxins.

Female sex has been linked to an increased vulnerability for AD, even after controlling for the effects of longevity. Decreased incidence has been demonstrated in women who have had oestrogen replacement therapy which has also been linked to improved cognitive performance in AD.

Psychological factors

Low educational level and poor linguistic ability have been reported to increase susceptibility to AD.[90] Confounding factors may be impaired nutrition or increased exposure to toxins, however those with higher educational level could have greater cerebral reserve and strengthened synaptic connections. Small head circumference which is a measure of brain size, is correlated with more rapid progression of AD.[91]

A history of depression is associated with an increased relative risk of late onset AD. This holds true for depressive episodes occurring more than ten years before the onset of dementia making it likely that depression is a true risk factor. Both depression and AD are associated with overactivity of the hypothalamic-pituitary adrenal axis with increased circulating levels of cortisol and non-suppression after dexamethasone. Raised corticosteroid levels have been shown to cause hippocampal damage in rats and primates which worsens with increasing age, and hypercortisolaemia has been correlated with rate of clinical progression in AD.[92]

Medical factors

Excessive microvascular pathology and blood brain barrier dysfunction have led to the implication of blood vessel abnormalities in the pathogenesis of AD. This has challenged the traditional division between AD and vascular dementia. Although there is a tendency for blood pressure to decline in the years immediately before dementia develops, the risk of subsequently developing AD is positively correlated with diastolic blood pressure at the age of 70.[93] In those with neuropathological criteria of AD, cerebral infarcts are more likely to be associated with clinical dementia.[94]

In mammals, experimentally induced diabetes leads to memory deficits and some data suggest that the consequent hyperglycaemia and hypoinsulinaemia could increase the vulnerability of neurons to damage by pathological events such as hypoxia, hypoglycaemia or Aß deposition.[95] Adults with maturity onset diabetes mellitus were shown to have a significantly increased risk of dementia (x 1.66), with the risk of AD more than doubled for men.[96] Hypothyroidism and epilepsy have also been linked to an increase risk of Alzheimer's Disease.[98]

Head Injury

Severe head injury involving loss of consciousness is associated with increased incidence of AD.[98] The risk may be greatest during the presymptomatic phase of AD in which the capacity for recovery is reduced. Post mortem studies following fatal head injury demonstrate an over-expression of the APP with the potential for increased deposition of Aß. NFT and senile plaques occur in the brains of boxers with dementia pugilistica, and Aß deposition is found in the brains of approximately a third of people who die after severe brain injury. A history of previous head injury and possession of an ε4 allele results in a ten fold increase in the risk of AD compared with a two fold increase in risk with possession of APOE ε4 alone, demonstrating a possible synergism between genetic and environmental risk factors.[97]

Toxins

Aluminium has been demonstrated in senile plaques and NFTs. It has been suggested that aluminium may enter cells and interfere with the production of Aß from the APP, induce aggregation of Aß and contribute to the formation of NFTs.

The EURODEM meta-analysis (1992) suggested a small reduction in the relative risk was associated with occupational exposure to solvents and lead. Although heavy alcohol consumption is linked to an increased incidence of dementia in general, it is not associated with AD and high alcohol intake may confer a slightly reduced risk. Similarly smoking has been associated with a decreased relative risk. When smokers were classified according to the number of pack/years (i.e. number of cigarettes smoked/day x years smoking) the relative risk significantly decreased with increasing number of pack/years ($p = 0.0003$).[98] There have been a number of methodological criticisms of these latter analyses including selection bias and inadequate control for confounding factors. Overall, a significant effect of toxins in the pathogenesis of AD has yet to be demonstrated.

DEMENTIA RISK FACTORS	
Age	
Female Sex	
Genetics	APOE Ɛ4genotype
	APP, PS gene mutations
Psychological Factors	Low intelligence
	Illiteracy
	Small head size
History of Depression	
Medical Factors	Cardiovascular disease
	Diabetes
	Hypothyroidism
	Epilepsy
Head Injury	
?Toxins	

Table 14

SUMMARY
Advances in the understanding of neuropathology have resulted in improvements in the diagnostic specificity and symptomatic treatment of AD. The next decade will be an exciting time in AD research as more effective treatments and primary preventative measures are anticipated.

References

79. Zubenko, G. (1997) Molecular Neurobiology of Alzheimer's Disease (Syndrome?). Harvard Review of Psychiatry; 5: 177-213.

80. Carr, D.B., Goate, A., Morris, J.C. (1997). Current concepts in the pathogenesis of Alzheimer's disease. American Journal of Medicine; 103(3A): 3S-10S.

81. Cummings, J.L., Mega, M (1996). Alzheimer's disease: etiologies and pathogenesis. The Consultant Pharmacist; 11 (suppl E): 8-15.

82. Guo,Q., Fu, W., Xie,J., Luo, H., Sells, S.F., Geddes,J.W., Bondada, V., Rangnekar, V.M., Mattson, M.P. (1998). Par-4 is a mediator of neuronal degeneration associated with the pathogenesis of Alzheimer disease. Nature Medicine; 4: 957-962.

83. Procter, A.W. (1996) Psychopharmacology of Alzheimer's disease. British Journal of Hospital Medicine; 55: 191-194.

84. Corder, E., Saunders, A., Strittmaster, W., Schmechel, D., Gaskell, P., Small, G., Roses, A., Haines, J.L., Pericak-Vance, M.A. (1993). Gene dose of apolipoprotein E type 4 allele and the risk of Alzheimer's disease in late onset families. Science; 261: 921-923.

85. Hsiao, K., Chapman, P., Nilsen, S. et al., (1996) Correlative memory deficits, Aß elevation and amyloid plaques in transgenic mice. Science; 274: 99-102.

86. Scheuner, D., Eckman, C., Jensen, M., et al. (1996) Secreted amyloid-ß-protein similar to that in senile plaques of Alzheimer's disease is increased in vivo by presenilin 1 and 2 and APP mutations linked to familial Alzheimer's disease. Nature Medicine; 2: 864-870.

87. Poirier, J., Deslisle, M., Quirion, R., et al. (1995). Apolipoprotein Ɛ4 allele as a predictor of cholinergic deficits and treatment outcome in Alzheimer's disease. Proceedings of the National Acadamy of Sciences U.S.A.; 92: 12260-12264.

88. Blacker, D., Wilcox, M.A., Laird, N.M., Rodes, L., Horvath, S.M., Go, R.C., et al. (1998) Alpha-2- macroglobulin is genetically associated with Alzheimer disease. Nature Genetics; 19: 357-360.

89. Pericak-Vance, M.A., Bass, M.P., Yamaoka, L.H., Gaskell, P.C., Scott, W.K., Terwedow, H.A., Menold, M.M. et al.(1998). Complete genomic screen in late-onset familial Alzheimer disease. JAMA; 278: 1237-1241.

90. Snowdon, D.A., Kemper, S. Mortimer, J.A., Greiner, L.H., Wekstein, D.R., Markesbury, W.R. (1996). Linguistic in early life and cognitive function and Alzheimer's disease in late life. Findings from the nun study. JAMA; 275: 528-523.

91. Schofield, P.W., Mosesson, R.E., Stern, Y., Mayeux, R. (1995) The age of onset of Alzheimer's disease and an intracranial area measurement. Archives of Neurology; 52: 95-98.

92. Weiner, M.F., Vobach, S., Olsson, K., Svetlik, D., Risser, R.C. (1997) Cortisol secretion and Alzheimer's disease progression. Biological Psychiatry; 42: 1030-1038.

93. Kilander, L., Nyman, H., Boberg, M, Hansson, L., Lithell, H. (1998) Hypertension is related to cognitive impairment. Hypertension; 31: 780-786.

94. Snowdon, D.A., Greiner, L.H., Mortimer, J.A., Riley, K.P., Greiner, P.A., Markesbury, W.R. (1997). Brain infarction and the clinical expression of Alzheimer's Disease: JAMA; 277: 813-817.

95. Messier, C., Gagnon, M. (1996). Glucose regulation and cognitive functions: relation to Alzheimer's disease and diabetes. Behavioural Brain Research; 75: 1-11.

96. Leibson, C.L., Rocca, W.A., Hanson, V.A., Cha,R., Kokmen, E., O'Brien, P.C., Palumbo, P.J. (1997). Risk of dementia among people with diabetes mellitis: a population based cohort study. American Journal of Epidemiology; 145: 301-8.

97. Mayeux, R, Ottman, R, Maestre, G. et al. (1995) Synergistic effects of head injury and apolipoprotein ε4 in Alzheimer's disease: a link between divergent hypotheses. Neurology: 45:555-557.

98. van Duijn C.M., Hofman, A. (1992) Risk factors for Alzheimer's disease: The EURODEM collaborative re-analysis of case control studies. Neuroepidemiology: 11 (suppl 1); 106-113.

Chapter 7
Neuroimaging in Alzheimer's Disease and other dementias

Z Walker

At present, a definite etiological diagnosis of dementia can only be made at histopathological examination. There are over 50 different identified causes of dementia. Over the age of 65 Alzheimer's Disease, vascular dementia and dementia with Lewy bodies are by far the commonest three. Neuroimaging allows in vivo study of the morphology and function of the brain, and may help in making a pre-mortem diagnosis; imaging is used increasingly, not only by researchers, but also by clinicians.

Brain imaging can be divided into structural techniques such as, computed tomography (CT), and magnetic resonance imaging (MRI), and functional techniques such as positron emission tomography (PET), single photon emission tomography (SPET), and functional MR imaging (fMRI). Functional neuroimaging methods can be further subclassified into techniques which measure cerebral blood flow, cerebral metabolism and neuroreceptors.

Most neurologists, geriatricians and psychiatrists agree that structural imaging of the brain should be performed at least once in the evaluation of a dementing illness. Chui and Zhang[99] showed, in a prospective evaluation of 119 patients referred with memory loss, that structural neuroimaging (MRI /CT scan), changed the diagnosis in 19% of the patients and the management in 15% of the patients. The main aim of structural imaging is to exclude any treatable structural causes of cognitive impairment, e.g. neoplasm, chronic subdural haematoma, hydrocephalus. In addition, imaging helps to distinguish vascular from neurodegenerative dementia, and different distributions of cerebral atrophy help to differentiate, for instance, fronto-temporal or other lobar degeneration from AD.

CT and MRI studies in Alzheimer's Disease, mild memory impairment and normal ageing

There are three types of change that can be identified on CT/MRI scans in patients with AD. These are generalised cortical atrophy, focal (hippocampal, temporal lobe) atrophy and white matter changes. Serial measurements of the hippocampal and medial temporal lobe atrophy have the most diagnostic power.

Medial temporal lobe atrophy assessed by temporal lobe oriented CT scans can improve diagnostic accuracy of AD to around 90%.[100] Although radiological evidence of hippocampal atrophy on CT or MRI scan supports the diagnosis of AD, there tends to be an overlap between atrophy associated with early stages of AD and atrophy associated with normal ageing. Acquisition of serial scans overcomes this difficulty as each individual patient's first scan becomes a reference point for further studies. Serial scanning with CT rather than MRI is cheaper, more available and better tolerated by most patients, but it results in repeated irradiation of the brain and the lenses of the eyes. Although this is not a problem in the very old, it has to be borne in mind in pre-senile cases.

Serial scanning with MRI offers substantial technical advantages by comparison with CT. Fox, et al[101] performed an automated image subtraction of two MRI brain scans one year apart in each of eleven patients with a clinical diagnosis of AD and eleven control subjects. The AD patients had a significantly greater mean rate of atrophy than controls (12.3 vs 0.3). There was no overlap between the two groups.

Hippocampal volume measurements may be also a sensitive way of detecting pre-symptomatic individuals. Fox, et al[102] described a longitudinal MRI study of seven asymptomatic individuals at risk of autosomal dominant familial AD. Over a three year period, three at risk subjects developed symptoms. Volumetric measurements of the hippocampal formation showed that asymmetrical atrophy (>5% difference), developed in these subjects before the appearance of cognitive symptoms (while still gainfully employed and with Mini Mental State Examination [MMSE] scores above 28/30). Verbal and visual memory measures declined in parallel with hippocampal loss.

Further evidence that hippocampal atrophy on MRI is already present in the very early stages of AD and at time of minimal cognitive impairment comes from De Leon, et al,[103] who showed that hippocampal atrophy was present in

78% of minimally impaired, 84% of mild and 96% of moderate to severe AD subjects. Controls showed hippocampal atrophy in 29% but there was a striking age dependence. In contrast, the cognitively impaired groups showed atrophy independent of age.

Another study of interest[104] followed a sample of 44 cognitively normal older adults for 3-4 years. One subject became demented and 13 cases developed mild cognitive impairment. Baseline MRI measurements of hippocampal formation size significantly predicted a decline in memory performance. These results indicate that hippocampal atrophy may be a risk factor for accelerated memory dysfunction in normal ageing. Although hippocampal atrophy is a very sensitive marker for AD, it cannot be used at present as an absolute diagnostic test, as extensive hippocampal atrophy has been shown also in PD patients with dementia (possibly fulfilling the criteria for dementia with Lewy bodies).

Compared with the consistently observed association between grey matter atrophy and cognitive impairment, studies examining the relationship between white matter lesions and cognitive dysfunction in AD continue to come up with inconsistent results. Clinical studies have shown that the presence of periventricular white matter lesions does not always correlate with dementia.

Pre-clinical diagnosis of AD using PET

It is now well established that patients with AD frequently have a typical pattern of cerebral glucose hypometabolism in the posterior cingulate, parietal-temporal and prefrontal regions and that these levels decline over time with progression of dementia, although this pattern is not absolutely specific for AD and can be encountered in diseases other than AD. Reiman, et al[105] used PET to investigate the cerebral glucose metabolism in 11 cognitively normal apolipoprotein Ɛ4 homozygotes (91% of Ɛ4 homozygotes develop AD by the age of 80), and 22 individuals without the apolipoprotein Ɛ4 allele. They found significantly reduced rates of glucose metabolism in the posterior cingulate, parietal-temporal and prefrontal regions, as previously found in patients with AD, providing "preclinical" evidence that the apolipoprotein Ɛ4 allele is a risk factor for AD.

Cerebral perfusion studies in AD

Compared to PET, SPET has the practical advantage of being more affordable and accessible, and so has greater potential to become a standard clinical tool.

SPET perfusion studies show, in line with PET studies, that the most characteristic abnormality in patients with AD is a bilateral reduction of brain perfusion in the temporo-parietal cortex.

A number of studies addressed the issue of the diagnostic validity of visual evaluation of SPET in AD. They came to differing conclusions. The only study that had autopsy as the gold standard, found SPET to provide useful information in the differential diagnosis of dementia.[106] SPET correctly predicted the pathological diagnosis in 93%, compared with clinical diagnosis, which was correct in only 74%. Although perfusion SPET was very beneficial in distinguishing AD from Jacob-Creutzfeldt disease and fronto-temporal dementia, it did not differentiate AD from PD or DLB. Likewise, Ishii, et al[107] found SPET of value in the diagnosis of AD among patients with dementia. The sensitivity of bilateral temporo-parietal perfusion defects for AD was 95%, but the specificity was only 56%, highlighting the fact that a temporo-parietal perfusion defect is not pathognomonic for AD. By contrast, Bergman, et al[108] found the sensitivity of visually evaluated SPET to be only 29% and the specificity 80%, and thus inadequate as a useful diagnostic test for AD. Explanations for these discrepancies might include the difficulty of comparing results obtained from different cohorts, with a variety of instruments and different data processing protocols.

Comparison of functional imaging with morphological imaging in AD

An important study employing the combination of a structural and a functional imaging technique and genetics is that of Lehtovirta, et al,[109] who investigated 58 patients with early AD and 34 healthy controls. AD patients were further subdivided depending on the number of apolipoprotein ε4 alleles. All subjects had volumetric MRI images as well as HMPAO SPET scan. In addition to confirming that patients with AD have reduced volumes of hippocampus and amygdala compared with controls, the main finding was that AD homozygotes for ε4 allele had the most prominent volume loss in the medial temporal lobe structures. All AD patients had the typical temporo-parietal hypoperfusion but the subgroup with only one or no ε4 alleles also had frontal hypoperfusion suggesting that AD patients differ depending on their apolipoprotein alleles.

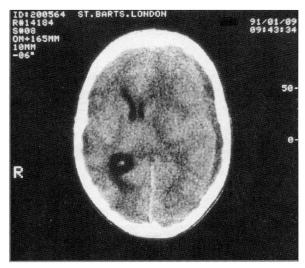

Figure 8
A CT head scan
showing a left
sided chronic
subdural
haematoma.
The haematoma
is hypodense by
comparison with
the brain. Note
the marked shift
of the brain to
the right.

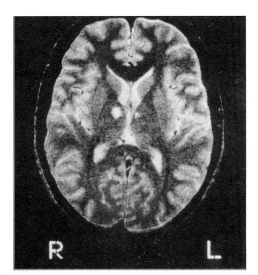

Figure 9
Bilateral thalamic infarction
in a patient with amnesia
but without dementia
(T_2 weighted MRI scan; the
infarcts show up as areas of
high signal).

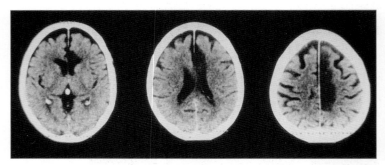

Figure 10. CT scans (three levels) showing a mature left anterior cerebral artery territory infarct. The infarct is of low attenuation and is seen starting anterior to the frontal horn of the left ventricle and extending up and over the lateral ventricle. The scan also shows frontal lobe atrophy.

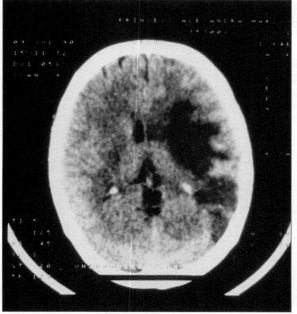

Figure 11
A CT head scan showing an early left middle cerebral artery territory infarct. The infarct has slight mass effect.

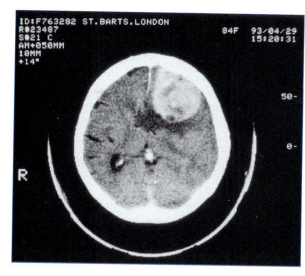

Figure 12
This contrast - enhanced CT head scan shows a large left frontal meningioma with some surrounding oedema.

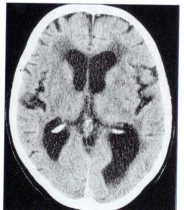

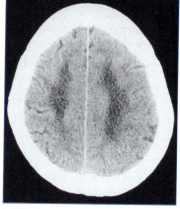

Figures 13 and 14 . The sort of CT scan which is difficult to interpret. Does it show hydrocephalus with periventricular lucencies, or does it show leucoaraiosis and central atrophy? It was reported by a radiologist as showing hydrocephalus, but the patient was hypertensive and had a mild, symptomatic gait apraxia and no cognitive impairment.

Vascular dementia

There are two sets of criteria that are commonly used in the diagnosis of vascular dementia *(Ninds-Airen & Chui et al).*[111] Both require the evidence of two or more ischaemic strokes by history, neurological signs and/or imaging, or a temporal association between stroke and the onset of dementia, or abrupt deterioration in cognition, or stepwise progression of dementia. Demonstration of an infarct on imaging is therefore mandatory for the diagnosis of probable VaD by both criteria. Although periventricular white matter lesions on imaging studies (particularly on MRI), are often interpreted as evidence of ischaemic disease, they can occur in normal ageing and AD and have not been shown consistently to be associated with cognitive impairment.

Dementia with Lewy bodies

Attempts to improve the accuracy of in vivo diagnosis of dementia with Lewy bodies (DLB) are important. Imaging techniques may be helpful especially in separating DLB and AD. Albin et al[112] reported on six cases of pathologically verified DLB studied with fluoro-deoxyglucose PET. In addition to the typical AD pattern of hypometabolism, DLB also had hypometabolism in the occipital association cortex and primary visual cortex. However Varma, et al[113] found perfusion SPET of limited value in the clinical differentiation of DLB and AD patients.

There is one preliminary report by O'Brien et al[114] that patients with DLB have less severe medial temporal atrophy than patients with AD.

One of the most challenging fields of research in functional neuroimaging is the in vivo study of neurotransmission. Dopamine D2 receptor ligands are now readily available and a number of studies evaluating their use in different types of dementia are in progress. Pizzolato, et al[115] studied the post-synaptic striatal uptake of 123I-iodobenzamide in 15 AD patients and in nine controls. They found that striatal D2 activity was reduced in AD compared with healthy controls. However, three of the 15 AD patients had extrapyramidal signs raising the possibility that some of their AD patients would have fulfilled criteria for DLB. Using the same ligand, Walker, et al[116] showed that clinically diagnoses DLB patients had significantly lower caudate/putamen ratios than either AD patients or controls. Further evidence that measurement of dopaminergic activity in the striatum may be of value in distinguishing AD from DLB come from Donnemiller, et al[117] who showed reduction in pre-synaptic dopamine binding using a beta-CIT ligand and SPET.

Fronto-temporal dementia

Fronto-temporal dementia (FTD) is a clinical syndrome characterised by a change in personality and behaviour with marked disinhibition, loss of insight, rigidity, perseverative behaviour, frequent affective and psychotic symptoms and severe impairment on frontal lobe neuropsychological tests. CT or MRI scan may show frontal and or temporal atrophy. Perfusion studies show a consistent bilateral reduction in frontal and anterior temporal blood flow which is visually distinct from that seen typically in AD, although not specific, as it can also occur in VaD and in AD. [118, 119, 120]

Conclusion

Imaging of the brain is contributing to our understanding of the dementias. At present its main usefulness is still as an adjunct to clinical diagnosis. With the increasing evidence that imaging changes precede the development of clinical symptoms, imaging of the brain may gain importance as an early diagnostic tool, and it may take on a role in monitoring the efficacy of different treatment strategies.

Acknowledgement

Figures 8-13 were kindly supplied by Dr RWH Walker.

References

99. Chui HC, Zhang Q. Evaluation of dementia: A systematic study of the usefulness of the American Academy of Neurology's practice parameters. Neurology 1997; 49:925-35.

100. Jobst KA, Hindley NJ, King E, Smith AD. The diagnosis of Alzheimer's disease: A question of image? Journal of Clinical Psychiatry 1994;55(11,suppl): 22-31.

101. Fox NC, Freeborough PA, Rossor MN. Visualisation and quantification of rates of atrophy in Alzheimer's disease. Lancet 1996; 348:94-7.

102. Fox NC, Warrington EK, Freeborough PA, Hartikainen P, Kennedy AM, Stevens JM, Rossor MN. Presymptomatic hippocampal atrophy in Alzheime's disease: A longitudinal MRI study. Brain 1996; 119:2001-7.

103. De Leon MJ, Convit A, George AE, Golomb J, De Santi S, Tarshish C, Rusinek H, Bobinski M, Ince C, Miller D, et al. In vivo structural studies of the hippocampus in normal aging and in incipient Alzheimer's disease. Annals of the New York Academy of Sciences 1996; 777:1-13.

104. Golomb J, Kluger A, De Leon MJ, Ferris SH, Mittelman M, Cohen J, George AE. Hippocampal formation size predicts declining memory performance in normal aging. Neurology 1996; 47:810-3.

105. Reiman EM, Caselli RJ, Yun LS, Chen K, Bandy D, Minoshima S, Thibodfau SN, Osborne D. Preclinical evidence of Alzheimer's disease in persons homozygous for the ε4 allele for apolipoprotein E. N Engl J Med 1996; 334:752-8.

106. Read SL, Miller BL, Mena I, Kim R, Itabashi H, Darby A. SPECT in dementa: clinical and pathological correlation. J Am Geriatr Soc 1995; 43:1243-7.

107. Ishii K, Mori E, Kitagaki H, Sakamoto S, Yamaji S, Imamura T, Ikejiri Y, Kono M. The clinical utility of visual evaluation of scintigraphic perfusion patterns for Alzheimer's disease using I-123 IMP SPECT. Clinical Nuclear Medicine 1996; 21(2):106-10.

108. Bergman H, Chertkow H, Wolfson C, Stern J, Rush C, Whitehead V, Dixon R. HM-PAO (CERETEC) SPECT brain scanning in the diagnosis of Alzheimer's disease. J Am Geriatr Soc 1997; 45:15-20.

109. Lehtovirta M, Soininen H, Laakso MP, Partanen K, Helisalmi S, Mannermaa A, Ryynanen M, Kuikka JT, Hartikainen P, Riekkinen PJ. SPECT and MRI analysis in Alzheimer's disease: relation to apolipoprotein E Ó4 allele. Journal of Neurology, Neurosurgery and Psychiatry 1996; 60:644-9.

110. Roman GC, Tatemichi TK, Erkinjuntti T, et al. Vascular dementia: diagnostic criteria for research studies. Report of the NINDS-AIREN International Workshop. Neurology 1993; 43:250-60.

111. Chui HC, Victoroff JI, Margolin D, Jagust W, Shankle R, Katzman R. Criteria for the diagnosis of ischemic vascular dementia proposed by the State of California Alzheimer's Disease Diagnostic and Treatment Centers. Neurology 1992; 42:473-80.

112. Albin RL, Minoshima S, D'Amato CJ, Frey KA, Kuhl DE, Sima AAF. Fluoro-deoxyglucose positron emission tomography in diffuse Lewy body disease. Neurology 1996; 47:462-6.

113. Varma AR, Talbot PR, Snowden JS, Lloyd JJ, Testa HJ, Neary D. A 99mTc-HMPAO single-photon emission computed tomography study of Lewy body disease. Journal of Neurology 1997; 244:349-59.

114. O'Brien et al; 1998; S205 p. Magnetic resonance imaging differences between dementia with Lewy bodies and Alzheimer's disease. Amsterdam: Second International Workshop on Dementia with Lewy bodies; Second International Workshop on Dementia with Lewy bodies.

115. Pizzolato G, Chierichetti F, Fabbri M, Cagnin A, Dam M, Ferlin G, Battistin L. Reduced striatal dopamine receptors in Alzheimer's disease: single photon emission tomography study with the D2 tracer [123I]-IBZM. Neurology 1996; 47:1065-8.

116. Walker Z, Costa DC, Janssen AG, Walker RWH, Livingston G, Katona CLE. Dementia with Lewy bodies: a study of post-synaptic dopaminergic receptors with 123I-IBZM SPET. Eur J Nucl Med 1997; 24: 609-614.

117. Donnemiller E, Heilmann J, Wenning GK, Berger W, Decristoforo C, Moncayo R, Poewe W, Ransmayr G. Brain perfusion scintigraphy with 99mTc-HMPAO or 99mTc-ECD and 123I-fl-CIT single-photon emission tomography in dementia of Alzheimer-type and diffuse Lewy body disease. Eur J Nucl Med 1997; 24:320-5.

118. Neary D, Snowden JS, Shields RA, Burjan AWI, Northen B, MacDermott N, Prescott MC, Testa HJ. Single photon emission tomography using 99mTc-HM-PAO in the investigation of dementia. Journal of Neurology, Neurosurgery and Psychiatry 1987; 50:1101-9.

119. Starkstein SE, Migliorelli R, Teson A, Sabe L, Vazquez S, Turjanski M, Robinson RG, Leiguarda R. Specificity of changes in cerebral blood flow in patients with frontal lobe dementia. Journal of Neurology, Neurosurgery and Psychiatry 1994; 57:790-6.

120. Talbot PR, Lloyd JJ, Snowden JS, Neary D, Testa HJ. A clinical role for 99mTc-HMPAO SPET in the investigation of dementia? Journal of Neurology, Neurosurgery and Psychiatry 1998; 64:309-13.

Chapter 8
Dementia rating scales

V Kirchner

Prior to the availability of potential treatments for Alzheimer's Disease, rating scales were seldom used in the clinical setting and usually only to screen for the presence of dementia or to roughly monitor change. Probably the most frequently used scales in clinical practice have been the Mental Test Score and the Mini Mental State Examination. More complex rating scales were limited to research and there was little need to develop these scales.

With the advent of potential treatments for Alzheimer's Disease, it has become more important to accurately diagnose dementia type and stage because treatments are generally aimed at subsets of patients. In an illness which has a natural course of gradual deterioration and which is variable, it is difficult to set parameters for outcome because lack of deterioration may be a good outcome, or merely the natural course for that person.

Pharmaceutical companies have also required sophisticated instruments with which to assess efficacy of new treatments. They require instruments that accurately identify patients with early Alzheimer's Disease and then monitor progression. The benefits of these treatments are often noted in particular aspects of function or behaviour, and if instruments are not refined, these benefits will be missed. This creates potential for instruments being designed to show a particular agent in a good light for commercial promotion. Pharmaceutical companies have been given guidelines on appropriate instruments with which to test their products by the European Agency for the Evaluation of Medicinal Products (EMEA), and the US Food and Drug Administration (FDA). The EMEA guidelines specify evidence of a statistically significant improvement in cognitive performance compared with placebo, plus either enhanced performance in the activities of daily living as measured by rating scales, or a global assessment of improvement made by an experienced clinician who is blind to other ratings.[121] Generally, the same collection of instruments are being used in trials of anti-Alzheimer drugs which means clinicians can become familiar with these.

Some rating scales are comprehensive, measuring many parameters such as, cognitive function, behaviour, motor function, activities of daily living, etc. Others are designed to only measure specific functions. It is often difficult to translate an improvement seen on a rating scale to clinical benefits.

Rating Scales can be broadly grouped as assessing the domains of cognition, global impression of change, activities of daily living, behaviour, quality of life, caregiver burden, and economics. Rating scales assessing caregiver burden and economics of anti-AD drugs are seldom used and there is a strong argument to include these when assessing new drugs. Examples of scales that could be used to assess caregiver burden include, the Camberwell Family Interview, the General Health Questionnaire and the Subjective Burden Assessment.

One of the most frequently used scales is the Alzheimer's Disease Assessment Scale-Cognitive Subscale (ADAS-cog).[124] This is an 11 item scale that specifically measures degree of cognitive impairment. Spoken language ability, comprehension, recall of test instruction, word finding, following commands, naming objects and fingers, constructional praxis, ideational praxis, orientation, word recall task, and word recognition task are assessed. The total score ranges from 0 to 70 with higher scores indicating greater degree of impairment. Normal elderly people may score as low as 0, although a slightly higher score is more usual. The expected yearly decline in AD is difficult to predict, but it seems to be in the region of 7-11 points per year, although in the earlier stages of the disease these changes may be greater.

The Clinician's Interview Based Impression of Change (CIBIC+)[126] is probably the most frequently used scale of global change. The 'plus' refers to the source of information including a caregiver as well as the patient. General, cognitive, behavioural and activities of daily living are the four areas of functioning that are assessed. Change from baseline is rated on a 7-point scale as follows:

1 = very much improved; 2 = much improved; 3 = minimally improved;
4 = no change; 5 = minimally worse; 6 = much worse; 7 = very much worse.

This method of rating is useful because it indicates whether change occurring in response to a new drug is clinically meaningful, and it more closely reflects the process that would occur in a clinical consultation.[126, 134]

The table below lists the most useful and frequently used rating scales in Alzheimer's Disease research.

SCALES OF COGNITIVE FUNCTION

Rating Scale	Abbreviation	Designed to measure	Source of information	Comments
Alzheimer's Disease Assessment Scale - cognitive subsection[124]	ADAS-cog	11 items of cognitive function are assessed: spoken language ability, comprehension, recall of test instruction, word finding, following commands, naming objects and fingers, constructional praxis, ideational praxis, orientation, word recall task, word recognition task	Patient	Clinician administers battery of brief individual tests (±1 hour). Score range 0 - 70 (0 = no errors, 70 = profoundly demented). Full ADAS has 11 cognitive and 12 non cognitive items
Cambridge Cognitive Examination[133]	CAMCOG	Evaluation of 8 domains: orientation, language, memory, attention, praxis, calculation, abstract thinking and perception	Patient	Maximum score 107 indicating no cognitive dysfunction. Cut off score for dementia is 79/80
Mini Mental State Examination[125]	MMSE	11 items of cognitive function including; orientation, memory, attention, naming, comprehension and praxis	Patient	Brief structured bedside interview (±10 minutes). Score range 0 - 30 (0 = severe, 30 = normal). Age and education effects. May not detect mild dementia, focal brain dysfunction or frontal lobe features

SCALES OF GLOBAL SEVERITY AND CHANGE

Rating Scale	Abbreviation	Designed to measure	Source of information	Comments
Alzheimer's Disease Co-operative Study - Clinician's Global impression of Change[134]	ADCS-CGIC	15 items assessed under domains of cognitive function, behaviour, social and daily function	Patient and caregiver	7 point scale: 1 = very much improved, 7 = very much worse. Designed to examine the process and determinants of making change scores
Clinical Dementia Rating Scale[128]	CDR	6 domains of cognitive performance assessed: memory, orientation, judgement and problem solving, community affairs, home & hobbies, personal care	Semi-structured interview with patient and caregiver	Global outcome. 5 point scale. 0 = no dementia, 3 = severe dementia. Total score range 0-18
Clinician's Global Impression of Change[134]	CGIC	Independent, multidimensional opinion	Clinician - based on all available information	General term for various measures of clinical assessment of meaningful change. 2 items: severity & change. 7 point scale: 1 = very much improved, 7 = very much worse. Clinicians vary in their opinions
Clinician's Interview Based Impression (Parke-Davis)[126,134]	CIBI	8 item scale including assessment of mental state, patient history, strengths and weaknesses, language, behaviour sensitive to change, motivation, activities of daily living	Patient and caregiver with a follow up interview with patient to assess change	7 point scale. Developed in co-operation with the FDA for tacrine trials

SCALES OF GLOBAL SEVERITY AND CHANGE continued

Rating Scale	Abbreviation	Designed to measure	Source of information	Comments
FDA Clinician's Interview based Impression of change[126,134]	CIBIC	Clinician's perception of change based on an interview	10 minute clinical interview of patient	7 point scale: 1 = very much improved, 7 = very much worse. Determines if effects of a given treatment are large enough to allow clinical detection
FDA Clinician's Interview based Impression of change plus[126]	CIBIC+		Patient and caregiver	Same as CIBIC except caregiver also interviewed
Global Deterioration Scale[131]	GDS	Global assessment of progression of disease cognitively, functionally and behaviourally	Clinician reviews all sources of information including patient and caregiver	7 point scale: 1= no cognitive decline, 7 = very severe cognitive decline
New York University/ Sandoz CIBIC+[126,134]	NYU CIBIC+	Semi-structured interview with patient (cognitive function and behaviour) and caregiver (functional activities and behaviour)	Patient & caregiver	7 point scale: 1 = very much improved, 7 = very much worse

SCALES OF BEHAVIOUR

Rating Scale	Abbreviation	Designed to measure	Source of information	Comments
Behaviour Rating Scale for Dementia of the Consortium to Establish a Registry for Alzheimer's Disease[136]	CERAD BRSD	8 factors map onto clinically relevant domains: depressive features, psychotic features, defective self-regulation, irritability/agitation, vegetative features, apathy, aggression, affective lability	Caregiver	Standardised, semi-structured interview
Behavioural Pathology in Alzheimer's Disease Scale[134]	BEHAVE-AD	25 well defined behaviours in 7 areas: paranoid and delusional ideation, hallucinations, activity disturbance, aggressiveness, diurnal rhythm disturbance, affective disturbance, anxieties and phobias.	Caregiver	Each behaviour is scored 0 - 3
Manchester and Oxford Universities Scale for the Psychopathological Assessment of Dementia[121]	MOUSEPAD	59 items of behaviour and psychopathology are assessed	Caregiver	Most items rated on 3 point scale: 1=mild, 3=severe
Neuropsychiatric Inventory[122]	NPI	13 behaviours	Caregiver	Structured interview. Score 0 - 120

SCALES OF ACTIVITIES OF DAILY LIVING

Rating Scale	Abbreviation	Designed to measure	Source of information	Comments
Functional Assessment Scale[129]	FAST	16 items of physical and instrument activities of daily living	Caregiver	Intended to project progression of loss of function in Alzheimer's disease
Instrumental Activities of Daily Living[127]	IADL	Assesses performance in the following activities: telephoning, shopping, food preparation, housekeeping, laundry, transportation, finances, responsibility for medication	Caregiver	Score range 6 - 30
Interview of Deterioration in Daily Living Activities in Dementia[137]	IDDD	33 item structured interview covering self care items and complex activity items	Caregiver	Frequency of assistance rated on 3 point scale for each item. Overall range 33 - 99 (99 = most severe)
Progressive Deterioration Scale[123]	PDS	Assesses activities of daily living including normal socialising, finances, awareness of time, walking without getting lost, remembering where things are placed, household chores, hobbies, use of tools, independent travelling, appropriate dressing and eating	Caregiver	29 items scored on a visual analogue scale 0 - 100 (0 = severe, 100 = normal)
Physical Self-Maintenance Scale[127]	PSMS	Assesses more functional or basic daily activities	Caregiver	Score range 6 - 30

SCALES OF QUALITY OF LIFE

Rating Scale	Abbreviation	Designed to measure	Source of information	Comments
Quality of Life	QoL	7 items evaluating feelings of well being including: relationships, eating, sleeping, social activity and leisure activity.	Patient	

References:

121. Allen NHP, Gordon S, Hope T, Burns A. Manchester and Oxford scale for the psychopathological assessment of dementia (MOUSEPAD). British Journal of Psychiatry 1996; 169:293-307.

122. Cummings JL, Mega M, Gray K. The neuropsychiatric inventory. Neurology 1994; 44:2308-2314.

123. DeJong R, Osterlund OW, Roy GW. Measurement of quality-of-life changes in patients with Alzheimer's disease. Clinical Therapeutics 1989; 11:545-554.

124. Doraiswamy PM, Bieber F, Kaiser L, Krishnan KR, Reuning-Scherer J, Gulanski B. The Alzheimer's disease assessment scale: Patterns and predictors of baseline cognitive performance in multicentre Alzheimer's disease trials. Neurology 1997; 48:1511-1517.

125. Folstein NF, Folstein SE, McHugh PR. Mini-mental state: a practical method for grading the cognitive state of patients for the clinician. Journal of Psychiatric Research 1975; 12:180-198.

126. Knopman DS, Knapp MJ, Gracon SI, Davis CS. The Clinician Interview-Based Impression (CIBI): a clinician's global change rating scale in Alzheimer's disease. Neurology 1994; 44(12):2315-21.

127. Lawton MP, Brody EM. Assessment of older people: self-maintaining and instrumental activities of daily living. Gerontologist 1969; 9(3):179-86.

128. Morris JC, Ernesto C, Schafer K, Coats M, Leo S, Sano M, Thal LJ, Woodbury P, Alzheimer's Disease Cooperative Study. Clinical Dementia Rating and reliability in multicenter studies: the Alzheimer's Disease Cooperative Study experience. Neurology 1997; 48:1508-1510.

129. Reisberg B. Functional assessment staging (FAST). Psychopharmacology Bulletin. 1988; 24(4):653-9.

130. Reisberg B, Borenstein J, Franssen E. Behave-AD: a clinical rating scale for the assessment of pharmacologically remediable behavioral symptomatology in Alzheimer's disease. In Alzheimer's Disease. Problems. Prospects, and Perspectives, ed HJ Altman, pp1-16. New York, Plenum Press, 1987.

131. Reisberg B, Ferris SH, deLeon MJ, Crook T. The global deterioration scale for assessment of primary degenerative dementia. Amercian Journal of Psychiatry 1982; 139:1136-1139.

132. Rogers SL, Farlow MR, Doody RS, Friedhoff IT, Donepezil Study Group. A 24 week double-blind, placebo-controlled trial of donepezil in patients with Alzheimer's Disease. Neurology 1998; 50:36-145.

133. Rosen WG, Mohs RC, Davis K. A new rating scale for Alzheimer's disease. American Journal of Psychiatry 1984; 141:1356-1364.

134. Roth M, Tym E, Mountjoy CQ, Huppert FA, Hendrie H, Verma S, Goddard. CAMDEX: a standardised instrument for the diagnosis of mental disorder in the elderly with special reference to the early detection of dementia. British Journal of Psychiatry 1986; 149:698-709.

135. Schneider LS, Olin JT, Doody RS. Validity and reliability of the Alzheimer's disease cooperative study-clinical global impression of change. Alzheimer's Disease and Associated Disorders 1997; 11(suppl):S22-32.

136. Schneider LS. CIBIC+: what, why and how? Alzheimer Insights 1997; 3(2):5-8.

137. Tariot PN, Mack JL, Patterson MB, Edland SD, Weiner MF, Fillenbaum G, Blazina L, Teri L, Rubin E.Mortimer JA. The Behavior Rating Scale for Dementia of the Consortium to Establish a Registry for Alzheimer's Disease. The Behavioral Pathology Committee of the Consortium to Establish a Registry for Alzheimer's Disease. American Journal of Psychiatry 1995; 152(9):1349-57.

138. Teunisse S, Derix MM, van Crevel H. Assessing the severity of dementia. Patient and caregiver. Archives of Neurology 1991; 48(3):274-7.

Chapter 9

Future treatments and the way ahead

V Kirchner

Up until recently, a diagnosis of AD was accompanied by a sense of therapeutic hopelessness. All that could be offered to patients and their families was emotional support, behavioural interventions and sometimes the use of psychotropic drugs to control some of the more troublesome symptoms, albeit ineffectively and with associated morbidity. Available treatments have increased and become more sophisticated. The benefit of memory aids and behavioural interventions are now well established. However, the real possibility of drugs preventing the onset or delaying the course of the illness has had a big impact on the level of interest that AD is generating. It has emerged from being neglected and poorly understood to being at the forefront of medical development. There is now the exciting prospect that in the foreseeable future AD will no longer represent a frightening prospect looming in old age, but a treatable condition. The potential to prevent this disease holds enormous cost benefits financially, and in terms of illness burden, which would dwarf the advantages of current symptomatic treatments.[139]

The management of AD in the future can be viewed in three categories:

- Primary prevention
- Treatment of established disease
- Treating complications and reducing disability.

Different potential strategies would apply to different stages of life (*Figure 15*) and these potential strategies are diverse reflecting the multifactorial aetiology of AD (*Figure 16*).[142]

PRIMARY PREVENTION

Diagnostic tests

Patients with AD have lower levels of Aß42, (43) and higher levels of tau

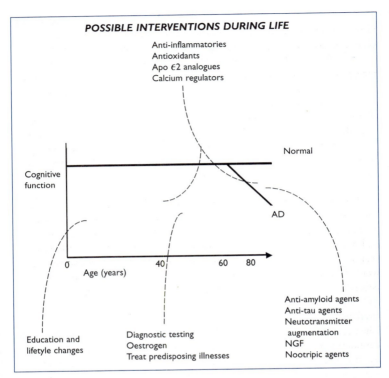

Figure 15

protein in their CSF compared with normal controls. They also have a protein called AD7c-NTP, which results from over expression of AD7c-NTP DNA. Tests have been devised using monoclonal antibodies that recognise these three proteins. The test identifying the presence of AD7c-NTP has high specificity (89%) and sensitivity (89%) for AD, compared with other dementias and normal controls.[140]

Genetic factors

Already, four genetic loci have been identified where mutations result in phenotypic expression of AD. The mutations on chromosomes 1, 14 and

21 affect a relatively small number of early onset cases and would be useful to identify individuals at risk in families with a known history of AD. For the general population, the presence of Apolipoprotein ε4 alleles may be useful in narrowing down those at greater risk. Not all cases of AD are accounted for by these genetic factors and the search continues for other relevant genetic loci. This information will become more useful as more effective treatments are available. At present, there is no point in testing individuals for genetic risk of AD as no curative treatment can be offered. In future, these test will be useful to identify individuals at risk so that they can be offered treatments that prevent onset of the illness. Understanding the genetic abnormalities help elucidate the biochemical abnormalities, and therefore, possible treatments can be explored to rectify these.

Lifestyle changes

Epidemiological studies have identified some lifestyle risks that can be modified and there is hope that (as in cardiovascular disease), these modifications will reduce the incidence of AD in the general population. Education, diet, exercise and protection against head injury have all been identified as modifiable factors that help protect against AD. A recommended diet of fresh fruit and vegetables would be rich in antioxidants. More risk factors will be identified and public education will inform individuals about modifying their lifestyles.

Predisposing illnesses

The occurrence of certain illnesses have been identified as increasing the risk of developing AD in later life. Depression, hypothyroidism, type 2 diabetes and hypertension, are all illnesses for which there are prevention and treatment strategies, and which should be recognised early and treated effectively as part of an overall approach to reduce the incidence or delay the onset of AD.

Risk modifying drugs

Drugs can also be used to modify risk factors. This is a well established concept in the prevention of cardiovascular disease, e.g. aspirin, lipid lowering agents. In AD, these agents would include oestrogen, anti-oxidants and anti-inflammatory agents.

Oestrogen

Women using hormone replacement therapy containing oestrogen have a reduced risk of AD.[150] This is unlikely to be an effect of confounding variables,

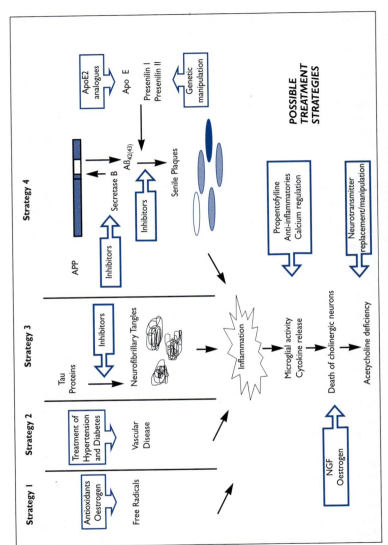

Figure 16

such as access to health care, nutrition and education as the risk reduction is highly significant. There are oestrogen receptors on hippocampal and cholinergic neurons. Oestrogen upregulates the activity of choline acetyltransferase and stimulates the growth of cholinergic neurons probably through increasing neurotrophin activity; particularly in the basal forebrain. It also decreases cerebral amyloid deposition, delays development of vascular disease and has antioxidant properties. Strong neuroprotective effects warrant serious consideration of oestrogen as a potential treatment. More prospective data is needed before oestrogen can be promoted as a risk modifying agent.

Anti-oxidants

Products of oxidative processes and reactive oxygen species, are known to cause neuronal membrane damage and induce amyloid aggregation and deposition. Superoxide dismutase is a natural free radical scavenger which, in AD, is found in levels reduced by 25-35%. The following free radical scavengers are candidates being investigated as potential treatments: selegeline, α-tocopherol (vitamin E), idebenone, tirilizadmesylate, and desferrioxamine.

Selegiline and α-tocopherol have been studied alone and in combination. Selegiline acts as an antioxidant inhibiting oxidative deamination, it increases levels of catecholamines and is an adrenergic stimulant. α-tocopherol acts by trapping free radicals. Both agents have a treatment effect of significantly delaying death, institutionalisation, loss of the ability to perform at least 2-3 basic activities of daily living, and the progression from moderate to severe dementia. They have no additive benefit in combination. They are both also associated with increased syncopal episodes and falls.[149]

Idebenone exerts antioxidant effects by enhancing mitochondrial adenosine triphosphate production. It also stimulates the synthesis of (nerve growth factor) NGF, and it protects against excitotoxic neuronal damage. Thus far, it has had only mild benefit in clinical trials.

Anti-inflammatory drugs

There is cytological evidence of increased inflammation in brains of people who died with AD including increased cytokines, microglial activation and complement deposition and activation. Epidemiological studies have indicated that individuals exposed to non-steroidal anti-inflammatory drugs (NSAIDs), have a lower risk of developing AD supporting the hypothesis that inflammation is important in the rate of disease progression. NSAIDs inhibit cyclo-oxygenase-1, which is induced by inflammation centrally and peripherally. Cyclo-oxygenase-2 is found particularly in limbic structures, including the hippocampus, and drugs targeting cyclo-oxygenase-2 are likely to be less toxic and more specific to the central nervous system, and therefore would be of greater potential use in AD. Colchicine has been shown to modulate the activity of microglial cells and it has some anti-amyloidogenic properties. Further evidence is required before long term use of NSAID can be recommended, as there is the possiblity that NSAIDs may precipitate agitated, confused and aggressive behaviour.[145]

Predisolone is currently being evaluated, but to achieve satisfactory anti-inflammatory effects, doses equivalent to 60 mg daily are required and in the elderly, adverse effects associated with such a dose would probably be unacceptable and limit its usefulness.

Apolipoprotein ε

The presence of apolipoprotein ε2 and ε3 alleles confer some protection against AD, as their function seems to be salvage and neutralisation of membrane lipids that have been liberated following tissue damage. This function is defective with the apolipoprotein ε4 allele, and this deficiency is potentially correctable with apolipoprotein ε2 analogues.[143]

TREATMENT OF ESTABLISHED DISEASE

Treating established disease could involve reversing the pathological effects, halting the decline of the illness, delaying the rate of decline or improving function.

Augmentation of neurotransmitters

Currently, the three drugs that have been licensed for use in AD are all CEIs which by inhibiting acetylcholinesterase increase acetylcholine levels in the neuronal synapses. Newer drugs with similar actions but improved efficacy and fewer side effects are being explored. Galanthamine, huperzine and metrifonate are three such drugs undergoing extensive clinical trials. Effects of these newer agents on domains other than cognition and behaviour are becoming apparent, for example, metrifonate may reduce apathy.

There is also evidence that drugs acting at the nicotinic and muscarinic type 2 receptors could be beneficial and these would be the logical successors to the CEIs. There is a deficiency of muscarinic type 2 receptors in AD. Drugs acting at these receptors that have an acceptable side effect profile have yet to be developed. It is also likely that they will be effective in only a subset of patients. Nicotinic receptors have been shown to be involved in learning, and memory and drugs such as, epibatidine acting at **α**4 ß2 receptor are being investigated for potential benefit. Nicotine itself has been investigated, but its propensity to cause insomnia limits its usefulness.

Synaptic transmission in the central nervous system involves a balance between cholinergic, glutaminergic and serotonergic systems. Thus far, research has mostly focused on the cholinergic system, but there is evidence that drugs like amapakane, a glutaminergic agonist, improves memory in normal individuals.

Ginko Biloba

Extracts from the plant Ginko Biloba have been demonstrated to have beneficial effects on attention and memory and are used in the treatment of AD in Europe. The differences in cognitive and social function seem to be sufficient for caregivers to notice however, they are not significant on clinician's global impression scales. It seems to have several modes of action including, protective effects on energy metabolism of neuronal cells under conditions of impaired oxidative phosphorylation, being a potent free radical scavenger, and enhancing choline uptake into acetylcholine producing hippocampal neurons.[147]

Propentofylline

Propentofylline is an adenosine uptake inhibitor that has glial cell modulating properties. Global function and cognitive performance are improved and the decline of ability to perform activities of daily living is slowed. These effects have been shown in mild to moderate dementia and they result in significant economic benefits. There does not seem to be a deterioration in function after cessation of propentofylline. It acts by inhibiting the proliferation of microglial cells, inhibiting oxygen free radical formation, inhibiting cytokine release and increasing the formation of NGF by astrocytes. Currently, it is undergoing clinical trials worldwide.[148, 151]

Drugs targeting amyloid and tau protein

The two pathological hallmarks of AD are senile plaques containing Aß and neurofibrillary tangles containing hyperphosphorylated tau protein. Aß is a less soluble form of amyloid. The enzymatic cleavage of amyloid precursor protein into Aß could be targeted by a future drug. Drugs targeting these pathways have yet to be developed. Possible modes of action include, inhibiting Aß forming enzymes, reducing the processing of amyloid precursor protein away from Aß, inhibiting aggregation and promoting dissolution of Aß, ameliorating toxicity of Aß and suppressing the reactive response to Aß toxicity.

Already eight protein kinases have been identified that are involved in the hyperphosphorylation of tau protein.[141] The potential for future treatments includes drugs inhibiting these enzymes or introducing enzymes that dephosphorylate tau protein.

Nerve growth factor

In experimental models of intracerebral administration of NGF, it has been found to enhance the growth and development of forebrain cholinergic neurons, particularly those that innervate the cortex and hippocampus. The shortage of human recombinant beta NGF, and the limitations of intracerebral administration, currently make it an impractical treatment option in the clinical setting. However, it is possible in the future that NGF is administered through implantation of NGF secreting cells.

Calcium regulation

Damage caused by glutamate and other neurotoxins is mediated by calcium entry into the affected neurons. Calcium influx is a critical step in amyloid induced neurotoxicity and regulation of calcium entry into the cell may limit this damage. Calcium channel blocking drugs, such as nimodipine, which have been shown in low doses in controlled trials to improve cognitive function and behavioural features in AD, may have a role to play.

Nootropic agents

Nootropic agents are also known as cognitive enhancers. Numerous agents believed to have cognitive enhancing properties have been investigated in the past including vasodilators. Most have shown some benefit in a very small subset of patients. Recent agents that have been investigated are piracetam, aniracetam, oxiracetam and paramiracetam. This type of agent may have a limited role in combination with other drugs.

Heavy metals
Heavy metals promote the aggregation of ß4 Amyloid suggesting that chelating agents such as chysramine, which inactivates these metals might have therapeutic application.

TREATING COMPLICATIONS AND REDUCING DISABILITY

Compensating for cognitive deficits
Interventions are becoming increasingly accepted and sophisticated. These include memory training, memory aids and reality orientation.

Caregiver support
The role and burden on caregivers is becoming increasingly apparent and supporting caregivers results in lower rates of institutionalisation and a decreased burden of care. In the future increased resources will be directed at caregivers.

Behavioural and environmental interventions
In the past, troublesome behaviours and symptoms have been targeted with psychotropic drugs. There is now evidence that particularly neuroleptic drugs are no more effective than placebo and they may hasten cognitive decline, so more emphasis is being placed on improved behavioural and environmental intervention techniques targeting these complications.

CONCLUSIONS
The most likely scenario of the foreseeable future in treating AD is the use of combination treatments of neurotransmitter replacement drugs with NSAIDs and anitoxidants. The efficacy and interactions of such combinations have yet to be tested. Oestrogen is also likely to become an important prevention strategy in women at risk. Drugs protecting against the toxic effects of Aß are still in early stages of research. Any drug treatment will be used in combination with social, environmental and behavioural interventions along with more sophisticated support for caregivers.

As more effective treatments become available, tests to identify individuals at risk will become more important including tests identifying genetic and biochemical markers of AD.

It can be expected that more reliable and efficient measures of clinically meaningful outcomes will be developed to test new treatments and to evaluate patient response to a particular treatment. Predictors of rate of decline, and factors identifying subgroups of patients sensitive to particular therapeutic agents, will also play a more important role in future care.

With the availability of modestly efficacious treatments, it is increasingly difficult to justify placebo controls when evaluating experimental treatments and these newer treatments may have to be tested as 'add-on' treatments. AD has multifactorial aetiology with genetic and environmental factors interacting in a complex relationship, modulating the risk of developing the disease. Major environmental risk factors have yet to be elucidated and once this happens, primary prevention will be more effective.

References

139. Brodaty H. Realistic expectations for Alzheimer's disease management. Therapeutic progress in Alzheimer's disease management. 9th European College of Neuropsychopharmacology, Amsterdam, 1996.

140. Ghanbari H, Ghanbari K, Munzar M, Averback P. Specifity of AD7c-NTP as a biochemical marker for Alzheimer's disease. Journal of Contemporary Neurology 1998; 4A:2-6.

141. Imahori K, Hoshi M, Ishiguro K, Sato K, Takahashi M, Shiurba R, Yamaguchi H, Takashima A, Uchida T. Possible role of Tau protein kinases in pathogenesis of Alzheimer's disease. Neurobiology of Aging 1998; 19 (Suppl.1):S93-S98.

142. Knopman DS, Morris JC. An update on primary drug therapies for Alzheimer's disease. Archives of Neurology 1998; 54:1406-1409.

143. Leonard BE. Advances in the drug treatment of Alzheimer's disease. Human Psychopharmacology 1998; 13:83-90.

144. Lethem R. Anitoxidants and dementia. Lancet 1997; 349:1189.

145. Mallet L, Kuyumjian J. Indomethacin-induced behavioural changes in an elderly patient with dementia. Annals of Pharmacotherapy 1998; 32:201.

146. Masters CL, Beyreuther K. Science, medicine and the future Alzheimer's Disease. British Medical Journal 1998; 316:446-448.

147. Maurer K, Ihl R, Dierks T, Frolich L. Clinical efficacy of Ginko Biloba special extract EGb 761 in dementia of the Alzheimer type. Journal of Psychiatric Research 1997; 31(6):645-55.

148. Rother M, Erkinjuntti T, Roessner M, Kittner B, Marcusson J, Karlsson I. Proprentofylline in the treatments of Alzheimer's disease and vascular dementia: a review of phase III trials. Dementia Geriatric Cognitive Disorders 1998; 9(suppl1):36-43.

149. Sano M, Ernesto C, Thomas RG, Klauber MR, Schafer K, Grundman M, Woodbury P, Growdon J, Cotman CW, Pfeiffer E, Schneider LS, Thal LJ. A controlled trial of selegiline, alpha-tocopherol, or both as treatment for Alzheimer's Disease. New England Journal of Medicine 1997; 336(17): 1216-1222.

150. Tang M, Jacobs D, Stern Y, Marder K, Schofield P, Gurland B, Andrews M. Effect of oestrogen during menopause on risk and age of onset of Alzheimer's disease. Lancet 1996; 348:429-32.

151. Wimo A, Witthaus E, Rother M, Winblad B. Economic impact of introducing propentofylline for the treatment of dementia in Sweden. Clinical Therapeutics 1998; 20(3):552-66.